Community Mental
Health Teams

Oxford Medical Publications

Community Mental Health Teams: A Guide to Current Practices

Tom Burns
Professor of Social Psychiatry
University of Oxford

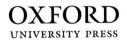
OXFORD
UNIVERSITY PRESS

This book has been printed digitally and produced in a standard specification
in order to ensure its continuing availability

OXFORD
UNIVERSITY PRESS

Great Clarendon Street, Oxford OX2 6DP

Oxford University Press is a department of the University of Oxford.
It furthers the University's objective of excellence in research, scholarship,
and education by publishing worldwide in

Oxford New York

Auckland Cape Town Dar es Salaam Hong Kong Karachi
Kuala Lumpur Madrid Melbourne Mexico City Nairobi
New Delhi Shanghai Taipei Toronto
With offices in
Argentina Austria Brazil Chile Czech Republic France Greece
Guatemala Hungary Italy Japan South Korea Poland Portugal
Singapore Switzerland Thailand Turkey Ukraine Vietnam

Oxford is a registered trade mark of Oxford University Press
in the UK and in certain other countries

Published in the United States
by Oxford University Press Inc., New York

© Oxford University Press, 2004

The moral rights of the author have been asserted

Database right Oxford University Press (maker)

Reprinted 2006

ISBN 0-19-852999-6

This book is dedicated to Eva Burns-Lundgren: a companion on this journey through community mental health care, and much more.

Preface

The last half-century has witnessed a massive change in Mental Health practice. The demise of the enormous and isolated mental hospitals which once formed the focus and professional cradle of that care has shifted and brought the mentally ill back into the mainstream of society. Some argue that this move has been essentially geographical and that the task of truly readmitting the mentally ill into society – ensuring equality of rights and social inclusion – is still to be achieved. Despite this it is undeniable that we now live in a society where the mentally ill are among us, and familiar to us on a daily basis. They are not shut away and forgotten in asylums about which we harbour simultaneous yet contradictory assumptions that they are benign caring communities and that they shielded us from scary and dangerous people. Few would regret the direction of travel of these changes although there are those who think they have been too rapid, and sometimes at a cost to families and wider groups that has been unfair. For many patients the outcome is not what we would choose for ourselves and often characterised by impoverishment and lack of dignity.

This is not a book about the policies of community care. There is no shortage of publications, both clinical and sociological, about the process of deinstitionalization and the closure of the mental hospitals, the assessment of population mental health needs, the economic impact of these changes and the short and long-term outcome of discharged patients in various countries. Nor is it a book about the theories of community mental health practice.

This is a book about Community Mental Health Teams. One undeniable fact about the shift to community care is that the hospital as the centre of practice has usually been replaced with some form of multidisciplinary team. These teams are remarkably consistent internationally despite often strikingly different health care contexts and even warring ideologies. On reading proponents of conflicting positions of mental health provision one would anticipate that there would be vast differences in their practice. Experience teaches otherwise. One is struck by how, in these opposing camps with strongly held and expressed contradictory ideologies, the clinical practices often only differ at the margins. I have sat in team meetings and spent time with ACT teams in North America where I have been hardly able to identify what was different from my own generic CMHT back in South London.

We are in an era of active change in how Community Mental Health Teams are being configured. After 30 or 40 years of slow and steady evolution, without that much reflection or writing about their characteristics, we now have high profile prescription of team structure and practice. The reasons for this much more interventionist and prescriptive position on mental health care are complex and they are touched upon in Chapter 1. They draw heavily on published research for their legitimacy. While it is flattering to academics to believe that their research influences government policies there are some problems. One striking problem with this research is that it has tended to be focused on the detailed differences between teams with very little attention paid to what they have in common.

Generic CMHTs

The exponential rise of mental health services research in the last two decades has led to a helpful increase in specificity in describing team processes and structures. A consequence of this has been greater clarity about specific models and with this has come an element of 'market branding' with high-profile product champions. Because nobody owns them, generic CMHTs have no product champion and risk being overlooked.

Most of the specialized teams are derived from the generic adult mental health team, and are refinements of it rather than completely new approaches. (This may not have been the case for Assertive Community Treatment in the US which appears to have developed in something of a local community care desert (Stein and Test 1980).) The generic CMHT appears to be more like a hardy and ubiquitous weed than a carefully chosen and planted flower. Wherever severely mentally ill individuals are well cared for outside institutions CMHTs arise spontaneously in a recognizable form. It seems that nobody needs to instruct doctors and nurses to work together with routine meetings assessing and monitoring patients and establishing links with GPs and inpatient units. It just makes sense. It happens without any great directive, and indeed, seems so far to have survived significant assaults.

This rather rosy view of CMHTs' spontaneous evolution is, of course, an oversimplification. There can be strong barriers, societal and professional, which prevent them evolving. What is striking, however, is that if these barriers are removed then the CMHT evolves without the need for prescription. There are very significant problems with CMHTs – as there are with any multidisciplinary working in mental health (Chapter 2). There have been many high-profile incidences where they have been badly run and dysfunctional and they have recently got a bad press.

Why this single-author book?

Given the current high interest in the configuration of mental health teams, it seemed sensible to try and describe current practice so that there could be a sharing of knowledge between practitioners. I was particularly keen that the relative neglect of the origins and functioning of the generic CMHT would be rectified.

Why, though, a single-author book rather than an edited one? An edited book would have been easier and quicker with chapters on each of the specialist teams written by their product champions. There is also the added advantage that those product champions are, quite rightly, recognized authorities in their area with years of accumulated experience.

I decided against an edited book for two main reasons. Firstly there is no shortage of them and anyone can quickly access the ground covered in this book by reading the relevant chapters in a small selection of them. Edited books are also sometimes unsatisfying – patchy in style and with contradictions between the different contributions unresolved.

The second reason was that product champions tend only to see the advantages of their approach, overlooking potential drawbacks. They also usually describe a level of practice that reflects their charisma and commitment to excellence, which the rest of us have little hope of matching. Cutting edge teams inevitably attract much more highly motivated and able staff than is going to be replicated routinely. Enthusiasts often describe what they hope their team is doing rather than what it is doing. Sometimes a well-informed outsider, prepared to spend time with the teams and ask all the naïve questions that an outsider can, may find out more accurately what is going on than those preoccupied with day-to-day practice. I was quite struck by the obvious discrepancies between what I was told was the practice and what clearly was happening in many teams I have visited. This was not 'spin' or deliberate misleading but the inevitable price of enthusiasm. I am sure a visitor to my team would find similar discrepancies.

I moved after 10 years as a generic CMHT consultant to running an Assertive Outreach Team for 10 years. It will be obvious from the above that I think they share more than distinguishes them. However, there are important differences in structure and function between the different CMHTs making them better adapted to different patient needs. It may be that I over-emphasize the similarities at the cost of the differences. I do so in a climate where generally the differences have been exaggerated. I am also unsure that we yet know *which* of the differences are important. It is far too common to assume that all differences have a profound impact when it is highly probable that some matter and that some do not.

I am particularly grateful to the specialist teams who allowed visits to gather much of the descriptive material for this book. They showed enormous generosity and tolerance. Professors Sashi Sashidharan and Max Birchood allowed us (myself and Mike Firn) to visit their crisis resolution/home treatment and early intervention teams in North Birmingham. Professor Tom Craig and Dr Paddy Power gave us extensive access to the Lambeth Early Onset team and Dr John Hoult to the South Islington crisis resolution/home treatment team.

They and their team members allowed us to observe their work at first hand and answered endless questioning. All of these teams have read the relevant chapters, contributed very helpful comments and clarifications, and have corrected mistakes. I thank them for making the book what it is but must take final responsibility for what is contained in the printed volume. There were issues where we simply could not agree – usually where practice differed from theory or where the differences in practice between teams meant that a course had to be steered between a faithful reflection of any one individual team. Dr Swaran Singh made many valuable contributions to the chapter on Early Intervention.

Personally I have found the whole exercise of visiting these teams and discussing their practice immensely rewarding – honest disagreement and recognition of variation is part of the pleasure of academic and clinical work. None of the minor caveats here about how the teams are cited should detract from the fact that they were all really out-standings services. If anything too good to be the final role-models for the rest of us.

I am also specially grateful to my colleague Mike Firn who went with me on these visits and whose experience as an Assertive Outreach team manager and training as a mental health nurse, meant that all the probing questions were asked, and misunder-standings, contradictions, and inconsistencies doggedly tracked down and resolved. Lastly, thanks need to go to my Personal Assistant Jerry Bowers, who has a remarkable human attribute of seeming to enjoy endless redrafting of my efforts and never loses patience with it (or with me).

Contents

CHAPTER 1

The origins of community psychiatry

'Community Psychiatry' is a slippery term. It is used widely, and generally with positive connotations, implying a more liberal and progressive approach to the care of the mentally ill. At its simplest form it contrasts the care previously afforded to patients for extensive periods of their lives in large, impersonal asylums with services that exist in a range of settings outside those walls. The simplistic story presented to medical students in the 1960s and 1970s was that the use of effective antipsychotics with the discovery of chlorpromazine in 1952 and haloperidol in 1958 'revolutionized' attitudes towards mental illness (Brill and Patton 1962). They brought optimism and therapeutic activity to what had previously been an essentially custodial function. From this, so the story continued, the move into the community began. Of course it is not that simple. Douglas Bennett (coeditor of an influential book devoted to the subject) comments that it is simply impossible to say with any conviction when community psychiatry as such started (Bennett 1991).

As we begin the 21st century, community psychiatry remains as controversial as it was in the 1960s, although the asylums with which it was contrasted with then hardly exist in the industrialized West. Still there are passionate and committed proponents of community psychiatry who compare it against 'institutional' systems (often comprising day hospitals and inpatient units in District General Hospitals) that only 40 years ago would have been considered models of progressive community care.

A 'heroic' view

A heroic view of community psychiatry based on this myth of a dramatic paradigm shift still persists. Among those psychiatrists who take a narrow biomedical view of the subject, the story is one of the liberation of patients by the discovery of effective medicines, which removed tormenting symptoms and permitted recovery and rehabilitation (Brill and Patton 1962). Among others, both within the profession and around it (particularly social scientists), the dramatic liberation comes from the triumph of a radical rethinking of deviance and its social control embodied in the 'anti-psychiatry movement' of the 1960s (Foucault 1965; Goffman 1960; Laing 1960; Szasz 1972).

Both these heroic visions have probably more in common than what divides them. They both emphasize an internal driver for change – it is the professionals (whether the professional doctor or researcher or the professional thinker) who made the difference.

Undoubtedly new treatments and new ideas (especially when eloquently and passionately expressed – Goffman's Asylum is *the* most frequently quoted text in academic sociology) have profoundly influenced the progress of psychiatry. However it would be misleading either to think of this progress as being mainly characterized by abrupt leaps, or to think that it is not related to broader social factors and developments.

Psychiatry has never stood still. There has never been a 'golden age' when the profession was fully at peace with itself, convinced that it had found the right approach and content simply to carry on. There has always been debate and dissent about practice. This should come as no surprise given the nature of a pscychiatrist's work, in particular the degree of subjectivity essential to a focus on the life of the mind. Psychology as a discipline grew out of philosophy, and philosophy has never tolerated absolutes for long.

External social influences

The raw material of psychiatric and mental health practice is human behaviour and this does not take place in a vacuum. It takes place between people and is first and foremost a social manifestation. Despite the wishes of some psychiatrists to locate the discipline squarely in biomedicine, it inevitably straddles both the biological and the social sciences. It is not possible to study human behaviour except in a social situation, or to make any real sense of it without some understanding of that social situation. Just as behaviour is studied between individuals much of its meaning is ascribed by individuals – the very nature of psychopathology is significantly socially determined. Changes in psychiatric practice have often been driven by social changes outwith the discipline. Tracking the development of community psychiatry demands of us that we take account of the social changes (both material and ideological) in which the care is located.

What is a cause and what is a consequence is not always that easy to distinguish. Some humility is needed in trying to follow the development of community psychiatry. We may think we see a pattern and draw conclusions, but need to remind ourselves that these are simply judgements. We are not in the position of natural scientists who can perform an experiment to resolve two conflicting opinions. In examining the rapid changes in practice in UK social psychiatry in the late 1940s I have tended to consider two forces particularly important – firstly, the establishment of the Welfare State and secondly, the impact on a group of unusually talented military psychiatrists treating stress disorders in soldiers. There is no way of knowing with any certainty that both did play a significant part. It is hard to believe that the subsequent developments could have occurred without the Welfare State. Whether the social psychiatry conceptualizations that arose from the Northfield experiment (Main 1946) and the Mill Hill unit (Jones 1952) were necessary for these changes, or materially accelerated them, or had no effect at all and were just associated in time cannot be *proved* one way or the other.

In short, the outline that follows is a story pieced together from writings and accounts which have made sense to me. The emphasis laid on individual events or factors is inevitably only one of several possible interpretations. The thread running through this brief overview is one that I think holds true. It is that trying to understand mental illness and the care of the mentally ill is driven both by society's more general values and ethics, and also by an increasingly confident application of scientific thinking (both in the social and biological sciences). So far I have used the term 'psychiatry' rather than 'mental health', and 'mental illness' rather than 'madness', simply to narrow the focus. The broader anthropological understanding beyond times and places where mental illnesses have been the business of doctors and nurses (and of course, often psychologists and sociologists) are outside the scope of this book.

The asylum era

The early part of the 19th century saw a wave of investment in the construction of large mental hospitals throughout the industrialized West. Institutions for the insane had been established long before these – most notoriously Bedlam in London, built in 1675. Pinel famously removed the chains from the inmates of the Bicêtre Hospital in Paris in 1793 and ushered in a drive for non-restraint. These enlightened views were echoed in the foundation of the York retreat in 1796. The thinking of the time was that mental harmony would be restored to the insane by a moral regime of respect and dignity. It would be tempting to draw a simple distinction between these institutions and the subsequent asylums by emphasizing the increasingly medical construction placed on the latter. It is certainly the case that asylums were conceived as places for recovery and had medical superintendents to run them. However it is striking how little medical thinking was involved in their genesis. The drive to build them came much more from civil libertarians who were concerned with issues of poverty and the imprisonment of the mentally ill and their vulnerability and exploitation in the common workhouses where they were then detained (Jones 1960).

Asylum building flourished in the mid-19th century and continued into the early part of the 20th century. Their scale and architecture attest to how serious the Victorians considered the care of the mentally ill to be, and they reflect significant investment. In an echo of current community care thinking, asylums were initially viewed over-optimistically (that most patients would recover given time and care). When this proved not to be the case then they were justified on improvement in quality of life for their inmates.

Early concerns

Even at their height, however, there were concerns about the approach. John Conolly, physician superintendent of the Hanwell asylum and noted proponent of the 'non-restraint' approach, cautioned against hospitalisation:

> ... confinement is the very reverse of beneficial for it renders permanent the temporary excitement or depression, which might have passed away, in actual insanity.

> (Conolly 1830)

Concerns about the deleterious effects of such large institutions were expressed long before Goffman's immensely influential treatise 'Asylums' (Goffman 1960), where he proposed the concept of the 'total institution'. Arlidge (who had studied with Conolly) wrote in 1859:

> … many asylums have grown to such a magnitude that, in these colossal refuges for the insane, a patient may be said to lose his individuality.
>
> (Arlidge 1859)

Conolly even went so far as to recommend keeping a note of new cases in the local area and monitoring them at home, initially weekly and then fortnightly.

Overcrowding soon became a problem in asylums. Bucknill in Devon opened a boarding house at the seaside in Exmouth in 1856 for some of his more stable patients. This move was stoutly opposed by local residents who eventually came to accept their new neighbours (Bucknill 1858). Is there anything that is really new! Overcrowding and neglect became increasingly a problem in asylums at the end of the 19th and beginning of the 20th century. Disenchantment with asylums at this time was often expressed in a desire for smaller, more treatment oriented and medically focused hospitals. The first psychiatric outpatient departments were opened in Wakefield Asylum and St Thomas' Hospital London in the 1890s to try and reduce admissions.

The 1930s and new optimism

The mental treatment act: 1930

A turning point in UK mental health practice was the 1930 Mental Treatment Act, which allowed voluntary treatment in mental hospitals for the first time. This act arose from a Royal Commission which had been established between 1924 and 1926 because of public concern about unacceptable conditions in mental hospitals. Until that time all inpatients were committed, so it represented a very significant change in culture. It endorsed a more medical approach to mental illness, stressing the relationship between psychiatry and general medicine and emphasizing the need for aftercare. As well as legislating for voluntary care it legitimized spending by local authorities on out-patient care.

New treatments

The 1930s also saw significant shifts in clinical practice. On the medical front two new treatments brought increased interest and optimism. ECT was introduced with remarkable effects in both severely depressed patients (who at that time had a high mortality rate from inanition), and in calming chronically disturbed patients. It was initially introduced in the form of cardiazol-induced fits because of the observation of the mood changes that followed epileptic seizures. The optimism from the impact of such a dramatically effective treatment was compounded by the success of malaria treatment for cerebral syphilis (a significant group in older mental hospitals with florid disturbances and a dismal outlook).

Malaria treatment had wide-ranging effects. Not only was it a 'cure' but it was a diffi-cult and risky one that required skill and careful management. Patients were often managed in medical settings and this helped bring psychiatrists and physicians closer together and emphasized the 'medical' nature of psychiatry. Managing these patients in medical settings (where the legal restraints did not apply) was often illuminating as they most often behaved well and cooperated with care, thereby raising the question of the need for their legal detention.

Adolf Meyer and the American School of Psychobiology

Adolf Meyer's influence on modern mental health practice has been profound although many now would hardly know his name (Lidz 1966). After training in medicine and neurology in his native Switzerland he moved to the US at the turn of the century and slowly rose to prominence over the next 40 years. His major contribution was to bal-ance the overwhelming dominance of hereditary explanations of mental illnesses and emphasize the interaction between the individual and their environment. He increas-ingly conceptualized mental illnesses (and their treatments) as dynamic, open systems with multiple opportunities for change. His approach required a detailed understand-ing of the patient as a whole individual – not simply as the carrier of a diagnosis. This detailed understanding was encompassed in the 'life chart' that he encouraged his followers to construct as part of a full assessment. He emphasised the importance of an individual's 'reactions' to the stresses and strains that life put on him.

Meyer was productive in other areas (hospital reform, treatment, teaching, etc.) but his lasting contribution has been this recognition that good mental health practice requires a detailed, intimate, knowledge of the patient as an individual. It may not be necessary to collect so much detail to arrive at a diagnosis, but then diagnosis is only a small part of an adequate assessment. At one time considered the most influential American psychiatrist of his generation, his influence has possibly been more lasting in the UK.

World war II and the origins of modern social psychiatry

Some important developments in social psychiatry did precede the Second World War. Querido established his outreach services in Amsterdam (Querido 1968) and day cen-tres for the mentally ill were established in Russia (Volovik and Zachepitskii 1986). However the changes that were to take place in the UK during and immediately after WWII have profoundly shaped the practice of current community care as it has evolved within modern welfare states.

Therapeutic communities

Wars have often had strange, unexpected effects on professions. It is not surprising that they produce significant improvements in engineering and physics as nations compete in a life or death race for technological superiority. They also, however, raise the status of behavioural sciences – rarely is it of such vital importance to make reliable assessments of people or to help them recover and get back to active duty. Psychological theories and testing methodologies were fast-forwarded in the First World War. National emergencies not only focus the mind but also result in the deployment of individuals in areas that they would not have chosen. Drafting individuals with quite different interests and temperaments into professions can unleash real creativity (the sort of result that universities strive so hard to achieve with cross-disciplinary courses).

Several of the psychiatrists who worked in the military hospitals brought to them fresh minds – free of sterile preoccupations with genetics and sectarian ideologies that characterized the profession at the time. Pessimistic, deterministic theories based on inherited degenerative disorders were also spectacularly irrelevant when faced with acute battle stress – severely disabling disorders in individuals from healthy families who only a few weeks previously were the cream of their generation. Fresh thinking was called for, and imaginative approaches required, to deal with these problems that clearly related to recent stresses and to the environment in which the soldiers had found themselves.

Mill Hill and Northfield hospitals

The rich mix of psychoanalytic thinking, group process and a commitment to instruction and education made the two military hospitals at Mill Hill and Northfield spectacularly creative. Tom Main, the psychoanalyst, and S.H. Foulkes, the group analyst, at Northfield applied psychodynamic thinking to the hospital itself. They realized that, just as the traumatic environment of the battlefield had made their patients sick, the environment of the hospital could be used actively to help them recover. Shifting their focus from an exclusive attention on the individual patient to the set of relationships around them, they experimented with manipulating these relationships to foster recovery. Emphasizing the impact of the unit itself as a healing agent (rather than just as a location for the healing process) Tom Main coined the term 'Therapeutic Community' (Main 1946).

Maxwell Jones, working at Mill Hill (initially on 'effort-syndrome', or 'soldier's heart' as this anxiety disorder was then called) developed these ideas in combination with a more direct and didactic approach. He became aware of the conflict inherent in being simultaneously the soldiers' officer and their psychiatrist. His evolution of the therapeutic community stressed the active learning that could take place between patients, and the importance of reducing the status differences that existed between officers and men if they were to have any understanding of each other and establish effective communication. After the war he continued to develop these ideas in the Henderson Hospital (Jones 1952), which became the first 'Democratic Therapeutic Community'. This was characterized by its four core principles of 'democratization, permissiveness, communalism and reality confrontation' (Rapoport 1960) which combined to provide 'residents' with 'living-learning' situations.

Both these developments imprinted on modern psychiatry the importance of the social context and of interpersonal relationships – in the genesis of disorders, in their recovery, and also in the treatment process. Despite the theories that surround them they were both intensely pragmatic developments and set the tone for British psychiatry for the next 40 years.

The open door policy and early social psychiatry developments

Open door hospitals

The pace of change established in WWII continued in the immediate post-war period. This was a time of intense political and intellectual fervour. There was a global belief that things had to be different and a faith in decent civil society to achieve such changes. In particular there was a commitment to greater civil equality and inclusion – whether that meant homes for all, the establishment of the Welfare State or recognition of the human rights of the mentally ill.

Perhaps one of the most remarkable developments is that the move to 'open door' care took place then, well in advance of the antipsychotic drugs that are often credited with making this change possible. Dingleton Hospital in the Scottish borders was the first mental hospital to open all its wards and run a comprehensive local service with no locked wards. This process was started in 1945 and was fully effective in 1948 (Bell 1955; Ratcliffe 1962). Warlingham Park and Mapperley hospitals soon followed suit. Interestingly both Warlingham Park and Mapperley had reintroduced locked wards before their closure in the 1990s but Dingleton never did. This may tell us something about the impact of continuing social change on mental health practice. Urban hospitals may have had to resort to more restrictive measures 50 years later when social consensus had diminished and the complication of psychotic illnesses with drug abuse almost routine.

Day hospitals

Reducing the isolation of mental hospitals was associated with early developments in forms of day care. Day centres had been experimented with in the Soviet Union in the 1930s (Volovik and Zachepitskii 1986) and the first mental health 'day hospital', the Malborough Day Hospital, was established in London in 1946 by the pioneering Joshua Bierer (Bierer 1951).

Day hospitals became a central plank of the planning for reprovision in the 1960s and 1970s. By the start of the 1980s there were 15,000 day hospital places available and only a fifth of them were used by patients who had recently been inpatients (Department of Health and Social Security 1984). They have been, in many ways, casualties of the successful development of the CMHT in the 1980s and 1990s. As CMHTs have become more effective, with greater resources and more reliable treatments, the role of day hospitals (once so obvious) has become less clear. How they overlap with day centres, for instance (Brewin *et al.* 1988, Catty and Burns 2001) will need exploration just as how they will cope with the rapid developments in community-based rehabilitation such as vocational counselling (Drake *et al.* 1994). Irrespective of the controversy that currently surrounds the place of day hospitals in the provision of modern community mental health there can be no doubt that (along with the establishment of inpatient units in District General Hospitals (DGHs)) they drove the community agenda forward for at least two decades.

The three hospitals study

Although attention was shifting in the 1950s and 1960s to developments outside mental hospitals they still constituted the main work place of most mental health professionals. Powerful evidence of the importance of social factors in the progress of psychotic illnesses came also from within mental hospitals. It was widely known that there were well run mental hospitals and poorly run ones, and that the condition of their long-stay patients reflected this. A benchmark study was conducted on three anonymous mental hospitals (they did not stay anonymous for long), and demonstrated that their regimes differed significantly and that the clinical and social functioning of their patients were closely associated with this. This 'Three Hospitals Study' was influential in demonstrating that even in schizophrenia (where the genetic contribution was not in doubt) the course of the disorder could be profoundly affected by the social environment, and in particular the level of social stimulus and care provided (Freudenberg *et al.* 1957).

Early outreach

At this time experiments were already beginning into providing care for severely mentally ill patients in their own homes. The first Community Psychiatric Nurses (CPNs) were reported in Warlingham Park hospital in London in the early 1950s (Moore 1961). They followed up, usually on weekly visits, schizophrenia patients who had been discharged from the hospital. In the US, Pasamanick even reported a controlled trial of nurse support for discharged schizophrenia patients as early as 1964 (Pasamanick *et al.* 1964). Home-based care for elderly patients was pioneered on the South coast in the so-called 'Worthing Experiment' (Carse *et al.* 1958). The UK developments took place within the context of a developing welfare state.

The welfare state

The Victorian asylums were built for the indigent mentally ill from the cities who increasingly had no family to support them and who otherwise would be homeless and destitute. Family support was, if anything, less available for the long-term mentally ill in the 20th century than in the 19th. The extensive shift from institutional care to community care that the second half of the 20th century has witnessed was only possible with the arrival of financial support for these individuals through the Welfare State. Provision of a minimal income, some housing and basic medical care was made available for all citizens across most of Europe in one form or another. In the UK it was centralized and monolithic with the establishment of the National Health Service in 1948 (promptly incorporating the mental hospitals, previously run by the county councils).

Early resettlement

The welfare state meant that individuals who had remained in mental hospitals simply because they had no families to look after them and no hope of being able to support themselves financially (and there were many) could be discharged. These early discharges were often very easy and patients settled quickly into life outside hospital with only minimal support. The time was soon characterized by over-optimism, and in the late 1950s many came to believe that the deterioration found in mental hospitals was entirely or mainly a direct consequence of living in them (Goffman 1960). The term 'Institutional Neurosis' was coined to describe this demotivated and demoralized state (Barton 1959). Simply changing the environment was considered a sufficient cure. Certainly for many of the early discharges this did seem to be the case. Not surprisingly these early discharges were those patients who were least disabled and as time has gone on the long-term residents in mental hospitals contain an increasing concentration of highly disturbed and disabled individuals whose resettlement, though possible, has required much more effort and support (Gooch and Leff 1996)

The interplay between social factors and treatments

I have focused mainly on social changes to try and balance the excessive 'march of progress' picture where psychiatric treatments are deemed responsible for all the changes in mental health practice. Undoubtedly the introduction of effective treatments was enormously influential. The arrival of antipsychotics in the mid 1950s has been one of the most powerful drivers of deinstitutionalization. It is not a simple cause and effect however. This fact is elegantly demonstrated by the sociologist Mangen (Mangen 1985), who traced the impact of the introduction of phenothiazines across Europe. He found, firstly, that the rate of increase in their prescription varied from country to county and secondly, that the impact of this prescribing (in terms of patients discharged from long-stay care) was significantly influenced by the local health and social care structures. He concluded that the impact was somewhat more marked in the UK than other European countries because the welfare state in the UK was comprehensive and well co-ordinated, thereby facilitating the benefits from the drugs.

The 1959 Mental Health Act

A Royal Commission into mental illness and mental handicap (the Percy Commission) was established in 1954 to enquire into the conditions in mental hospitals. The commission arose out of a growing concern over the overcrowding and squalor in these institutions (just as in the 1920s). At their height at this time there were 150,000 patients in UK mental hospitals and 500,000 in the US. The commission submitted its report in 1957 and the result of their deliberations became the 1959 Mental Health Act (MHA).

This was a remarkably forward-looking act, and very enlightened for its time. It required those detaining the mentally ill in hospital to give clear reasons for it and to review it at regular, specified intervals. It allowed patients to be compulsorily treated, not just to avoid danger but in the interests of their health. Absence of this 'health' indication in some countries results in inconsistent and inadequate treatment of the most vulnerable individuals.

Continuity of care and social care

Even more radical, the 1959 MHA made two provisions which have established UK mental health services in their current form. Firstly it required hospitals which detained involuntary patients to provide outpatient follow-up for them. In effect this means that there is at least some minimal continuity of care across inpatient and community care with essentially the same staff remaining responsible for the patient at differing phases of his or her illness. This is still rare internationally where inpatient teams are often independent of community services (Chapter 8).

Secondly it legislated for involvement of local authority social services in the care of the mentally ill. Social services were empowered to spend money on the aftercare of the mentally ill and acquired a key role in the whole process of compulsory admission. Social workers in the UK make the application for admission (substituting for the family) based on the opinions of the doctors. Not only does this safeguard the patient's rights but it also ensures that social workers and social factors are kept in view for doctors. Specialized psychiatric social workers were very rare in the 1950s – there were only 8 in England in 1957 and this had risen to 24 in 1959.

The 1959 MHA produced major changes in UK mental health practice. The number of detained patients in the 1960s had shrunk to a tenth of the number in the 1950s (Bennett 1991). A measure of its forward-thinking is that the 1983 MHA is hardly different from its predecessor apart from some of the monitoring mechanisms. It is now beginning to show signs of age, however, and will soon be overhauled.

Deinstitutionalization

From the mid 1950s to the mid 1990s the number of inpatients in mental hospitals fell to a third across the industrialized world (with a few exceptions such as Japan and Belgium). The start time and rate of fall has varied across countries. The start was early in the UK and the rate of reprovision relatively sustained. In the US deinstitutionalization started somewhat later but progressed significantly faster. Because of poorer social care and accommodation provision the rapid closure of US mental hospitals (many of which were much bigger than their UK equivalents with inpatient numbers of 3000–4000) rapidly resulted in conspicuous vagrancy and shameful neglect (Talbott *et al.* 1987).

Italy

Italy ushered in its programme of mental health reforms and deinstitutionalization in style under the banner of 'Psichiatrica Democratica', led by the charismatic psychiatrist Franco Bassaglia and his politician wife. Law 180 in 1978 'abolished' mental hospitals and lead to their rapid closure (Fioritti *et al.* 1997; Mangen 1989). The Italian reforms have probably attracted most attention internationally. Not surprisingly, as with any major social change, they have been more successful in some regions than others and have received a mixed press from the establishment (Jones and Poletti 1985; Tansella 1987). Overall, however, the Italian mental health reforms seem now to be well-implemented and successful (de Girolamo *et al.* 2002). Certainly it is one of the countries which has been most successful in bringing the general population along with its reforms.

Germany

Widespread reforms in Germany have been less dramatic – in part because of the federal structure which requires extensive local decision-making. A national survey of mental health care (the Enquête) was published in 1975 and laid the foundations for subsequent reforms. It emphasized the establishment of DGH units and local, more flexible outpatient services (Bauer *et al.* 2001). The number of patients has halved from the 1960s and psychiatric hospitals reduced in average size from 1200 patients to between 200–400. Despite establishing over 160 DGH units, only one psychiatric hospital has closed altogether. Since 1989, German psychiatry has been grappling with issues of unification of two quite disparate systems (East and West).

The 'water-tower speech'

Initially deinstitutionalization was driven entirely by professionals within the service. There was strong political support as evidenced by Enoch Powell's famous 'Water-Tower Speech' delivered in 1961:

> This is a colossal undertaking, not so much in the new physical provision which it involves, as in the sheer inertia of mind and matter which it requires to be overcome. There they stand, isolated, majestic, imperious, brooded over by the gigantic water-tower and chimney combined, rising unmistakable and daunting out of the countryside – the asylums which our forefathers built with such immense solidity to express the notions of their day. Do not for a moment underestimate their powers of resistance to our assault.
>
> (National Association for Mental Health 1961)

Soon the moral force behind Powell's endorsement of deinstitutionalization was strengthened (perhaps even replaced) by a recognition of the potential financial savings of closing mental hospitals. Leona Bachrach has referred to deinstitutionalization in the US as:

> ... an unholy alliance between therapeutic liberals and fiscal conservatives ...

(Bachrach 1997)

Whatever the main driving forces behind this 'unholy alliance' the decarceration of the mentally ill caught the mood of the times and has reflected current ethical concerns with the civil rights of the mentally ill. As societies have become richer and more secure, the concerns of their inhabitants have moved on from simple material needs (food and shelter and safety from exploitation) to individual freedom and self-determination. As we value these issues more for ourselves (taking the more basic needs for granted) we value them for those we care for and they have now become prominent. Where an individual insists on their freedom and self-determination (even at the risk of comfort and security) we usually recognize and endorse the trade off – it is 'what we would do ourselves'. So it is that as deinstitutionalization has progressed many patients have found themselves living lives in society that may provide them with less physical comfort and ease than was available in better mental hospitals (a clean, warm bed, regular meals and laundry etc.). Undoubtedly, however, the vast majority prefer it. Few want to return and most, when specifically asked, report an overall raised quality of life (Anderson *et al.* 1993).

Different countries have followed different paths with deinstitutionalization – the Italians closed the 'front door' – provided small DGH inpatient units and redesignated their mental hospitals as they withered. The British and Americans emphasized the reprovision for long-stay patients first, and only later developed alternative approaches for routine admissions. The end result has been essentially similar with most large mental hospitals either closed or down-sized with refurbished and redirected accommodation. Indeed it is an interesting question whether a range of mental health inpatient provisions which are sited in the grounds and buildings of an old mental hospital are still 'a mental hospital'. More important than the buildings, however, is what has happened to the patients.

Deinstitutionalization of increasingly disabled patients

Where psychiatric units do contain long-stay patients these are a very different group to those who originally filled the wards of the vast mental hospitals. Now they are highly disabled individuals, invariably with persisting positive symptoms and also usually with severe behavioural problems. It is these behavioural symptoms (assaultativeness, sexual provocation, and impulsive behaviour etc.) that make it impossible to support them in more public settings. Nursing such patients humanely is a challenging task. It requires continuously balancing patients legitimate wishes and rights for freedom and flexibility with the obvious, and severe, risks to which they are exposed and which they can pose. Staffing inpatient services is, not surprisingly, increasingly difficult.

The TAPS study

Just as the inpatients in shrinking mental hospitals are an increasingly disabled and unwell group, so are those who are being reprovided for in the community. There are no 'easy' inpatients any longer – all the easy ones were discharged in the first waves. The Team for Assessment of Psychiatric Services (TAPS) project in North London has followed closely the reprovision for two large mental hospitals (Leff 1997). It was clearly not ethical to randomize patients to staying or leaving but a clever system was developed of firstly identifying the cohort of patients that the staff considered most appropriate for reprovision and then dividing them into 'stayers' and 'leavers' where the stayers were to be reprovided for in the next wave (i.e. a year later). With this methodology several hundred patients had detailed baseline assessments of clinical and social functioning data conducted and repeated at intervals up to 5 years from discharge.

This enormously rich database provided a remarkable insight into long-stay hospital populations and also staff attitudes. By the time of the study (the 1980s) the first wave of easy deinstitionalization had already occurred and it is sobering to read just how ill these 600 patients were. Certainly the stereotype of an asymptomatic 'burnt-out' individual simply suffering from institutional neurosis takes a severe beating. These were actively ill and often distressed people with multiple needs and disabilities.

The TAPS project provided a firm platform with which to answer many of the questions about the fate of individuals discharged from mental hospitals. It provides a powerful balance to the anecdotes and myths that usually define much of the debate on community care. Few patients were readmitted permanently (although many had acute admissions just in the same way that non ex-long-stay patients do), virtually all preferred being out (although few had initially sought it), and almost none were lost to follow-up or became vagrant (Dayson 1993). The TAPS project also demonstrated that there was a small number of patients for whom non-institutional care was simply not an option.

The hope that community care would be cheaper than institutional care was also tested in this study. There is no simple answer to this question. A careful analysis of the costs for individual patients demonstrated that different types of care were more cost effective than others (e.g. medium sized hostels rather than very small or very big, privately run hostels and supported accommodation rather than those that are council run). More importantly, while community care was cheaper for less disabled patients this was not so for the more severely disabled for whom community care could, in fact, be significantly more expensive (Knapp *et al.* 1990). Overall the cost of community care was calculated as less than keeping the two hospitals open.

Stigma and resistance to community care

A major challenge facing patients discharged from long-stay hospitals (in common with all other psychiatric patients) is their reception by a society which has been sheltered from the realities of mental illness for several generations. The asylums generated an 'out of sight, out of mind' attitude to mental illness. Lack of exposure to the realities of mental illness has generated fantasies and myths. Contradictory fantasies can, and do, coexist.

There is the unrealistic expectation that everything can be cured, which can result in anger from families and neighbours when patients remain unwell or deteriorate. The general population well recognizes that not all physical illnesses respond to treatment and doctors are not held accountable for chronic asthma or diabetes in the way they are for the limitations of mentally ill individuals. Nor is every death during surgery assumed to be the fault of the surgeon in the way that every homicide by a mentally ill individual is automatically assumed to represent a system failure. This poor under-standing of the limitations of care and the cause of mental illnesses is not surprising, given how little real *experience* our generation has of it. We have not grown up with it as we have with diabetes or even dementia.

These unrealistic fantasies of therapeutic omnipotence go hand in hand with exag-gerated fears of the dangerousness of the mentally ill and their chronicity (and thereby predictability). Both these exaggerated responses to mental illness have been further fostered by a more general culture of consumerism and blame. In societies which are fast losing their dependent stance to professionals and where individuals (quite rightly) expect more and more to be treated as involved equals in the interaction, there is an emphasis on checking that the care received is the best. Expectations have been raised and this has generally raised the standards of professionals. However, continually set-ting that standard just above the average means that there is likely to be a constant level of dissatisfaction with services.

The complex picture of assessing risks and benefits in a particular case can be diffi-cult to explain to individuals who experience only the patient they know. For instance, how do you explain the need to tolerate poor compliance with treatment for extended periods because you know that pushing for better compliance will result in disengage-ment and no compliance? Where previously these judgements were 'left to the profes-sionals' they are no longer. A cumbersome and long-winded bureaucratic complaints process only makes a difficult task more so.

Public fears of violence and danger

Fantasies about dangerousness have become a major problem for the mentally ill and their carers in the UK (more so than most countries). High-profile mandatory inquiries into any homicide by a mentally ill individual (including those whose disor-ders are personality disorders or substance abuse) if receiving care from specialist mental health services have been imposed since the tragic killing of Jonathan Zito (Ritchie 1994). These inquiries attract considerable media coverage and ensure that each tragedy is brought to the public attention on at least three occasions – the crime itself, the court case and verdict and then the subsequent publication of the enquiry. Apart from the debate about whether or not this process is useful, and for whom, it is clear that the public now have a seriously distorted view of the risk of violence from the mentally ill. It is currently believed that we are the victims of an epidemic of such attacks and that the cause is the failure to keep such individuals in hospital.

There is no denying that violence is associated with mental illness – it always has been. The likelihood of violence from psychotic individuals is about four times that of non-psychotic individuals (Noffsinger and Resnick 1999), and enthusiastic community psychiatrists must take some responsibility for having played this down. However the risks are small compared to general risk factors for violent behaviour (young, male, and abusing alcohol being the most obvious) (Coid 1996; Steadman et al. 1998).

There is really no evidence at all that community care has lead to a rise in homicide or violence by the mentally ill. On the contrary Taylor and Gunn have convincingly demonstrated that homicides by the mentally ill have remained remarkably constant throughout the era of community care while the rates for homicide by non mentally ill individuals has risen steadily (Taylor and Gunn 1999). As a proportion of homicides they have fallen.

Public understanding of mental illness and stigma campaigns

There is nothing new about stigma. It is often proposed rather romantically that older stable communities attributed spiritual qualities to the mentally ill and from this they acquired protection and status within those groups. The case of Julius Caesar's epilepsy is regularly quoted. Even a moderately brief visit to Asia or Africa will soon dispel such a rosy view. Certainly the mentally ill are often well cared for within their families and when non-disruptive can be tolerated within communities and receive charity. The more severely mentally ill do not, however, fare well. Particularly in the area of marriage (an essential, practical institution in cultures without a developed welfare state) they are profoundly discriminated against. If they become detached from their families in these cultures, social exclusion is often harsh and sometimes fatal.

Stigma is not solely reserved for mental illnesses. Chronic and disabling disorders, especially when they are poorly understood and particularly when associated with social disadvantage attract stigma. As disorders become better understood, and even more when there are effective treatments, the stigma attached to them diminishes. Two vivid examples are leprosy and tuberculosis. Both still attract considerable stigma in much of the developing world but TB has been rapidly losing stigma because of effective treatments. AIDS generates profound stigma in the developing world where the reluctance of patients and families to acknowledge the illness frustrates public health initiatives. AIDS is still stigmatized in the West to a lesser extent despite extensive publicity campaigns. Three common themes from the successful reduction of stigma in physical illnesses help inform our attack on it in mental illnesses.

Improving basic knowledge about the illnesses

Stigma is strongly driven by fear – fear of the consequences of a disorder and fear of the consequences of contact with that disorder. In TB and leprosy the fear was mainly of contagion and as the very low levels of infectivity were established and publicized stigma reduced. The fears about mental illness are usually about violence and upsetting behaviour. Schizophrenia is often still referred to as a 'split personality', and equated in the public mind with Jeckyll and Hyde and with rapid shifts to unpredictable violent behaviour. Mental health professionals are often quite unaware of just how little the general public know about mental illnesses. Even general health care staff can be surprisingly uninformed. A study of nurses working in general practice found levels of understanding of schizophrenia little different from the general population (Millar *et al.* 1999).

Psychoanalysts have suggested that most of us fear madness because it resonates with the unreasonable (the 'mad') within us that we deal with everyday. While we know rationally that madness is not contagious, we fear that some of the behaviour we see is too close for comfort to impulses and wishes that we routinely keep under control. For this reason we avoid exposure and emphasize the difference between us and those who are ill to reassure ourselves. There is probably an important grain of truth in this – our empathy with the mentally ill comes from the recognition of similar experiences in ourselves. It is this which makes us able to help, but may also make us wary.

Increasing knowledge about treatments

There are currently several national and international programmes underway to combat stigma against the mentally ill. Countries such as Norway and Australia have been in the vanguard but India has several innovative programmes raising public awareness about the reality of mental illness (both aimed at reducing stigma and also at encouraging affected individuals to come forward for treatment). In both Norway and Australia these campaigns have been associated with a drive for earlier recognition of psychosis (particularly schizophrenia) in the belief that earlier intervention will prevent some of the disabilities associated with the disease and produce a better long-term outcome (see Chapter 5).

Even in highly developed countries understanding and recognition of mental illness as that (mental illness, not irresponsibility or recklessness) is low. Using vignettes of a depressive episode and of a schizophrenic breakdown, Jorm and his colleagues demonstrated how low the public recognition of these disorders was (Jorm *et al.* 1997*a*; Jorm 2000). Generally the public recognized schizophrenia as a disorder more than they did depression. This study has been repeated in several countries with similar results (e.g. Switzerland (Lauber and Rossler 2001), Germany and Austria (Jorm *et al.* 2000)).

Increasing understanding of treatments

The second theme in reducing the stigma of mental illness is to remove the sense of doom and incurability traditionally associated with it. This means improving public understanding of the treatments on offer and what they can deliver. The Australian national campaign provided the opportunity to conduct a detailed survey of what people thought were the most helpful interventions with depression and schizophrenia

(Jorm *et al.* 1997*b*). Medical interventions were very low down the list preceded by psychological and 'lifestyle' interventions including 'getting out more' and diet. Compared to mental health staff the public consistently favoured such life style interventions for both disorders and for schizophrenia particularly favoured reading self-help books (Jorm *et al.* 1997*c*).

A greater understanding of treatments – what they are, how they work, what can be expected from them, what their side-effects are – helps one to understand the illness and to form a more realistic sense of the prognosis. For most of the general public, theories of how diseases are caused is of little importance but understanding how the treatment works helps focus on the disease and form a 'picture' of the process. Understanding how antibiotics treat a chest infection moves the attention away from the cough to an understanding of germs and infection. Understanding the difference between antipsychotics and antidepressants is a start in distinguishing different mental health disorders. They give an easier introduction to the basic principles of the disorders and treatments as we understand them (e.g. over-arousal and distractibility in psychoses, or tension, preoccupation, and poor sleep in depression).

Better understanding about treatments also helps destigmatize those caring for the patient, and indirectly the patient themselves. The vast majority of the population still routinely think of antipsychotics (and antidepressants) as sedatives and tranquillizers. They are seen as simply ways of calming the patient down, not treating an illness. The implication of this (though rarely voiced as such) is that the drugs are essentially ineffective and just a way of keeping the patient quiet while they recover (or not) in their own time. It also paints the psychiatrist as more concerned with keeping the lid on things than actively working with a patient to get relief from a distressing condition.

Distinguishing discrete disorders

Focusing on treatments also helps distinguish disorders. Effective antistigma campaigns have learnt that they must focus on specific diseases to make progress – not on broad groups of diseases. This is both because they need to raise awareness and improve knowledge before they can modify attitudes and behaviour and also because it just seems that most of us respond poorly to vague concepts and exhortations to be better people. So campaigns need to target depression or schizophrenia or Alzheimer's disease, not 'mental illness'. The same strategy is clear in cancer charities which run parallel drives for example for breast cancer, bowel cancer, leukaemia etc. It helps focus and identification and is not too overwhelming.

Exposure and disclosure

The third theme in effective anti-stigma (or anti-discrimination) campaigns is to publicise real-life experience of disorders. People need to recognize and get to know individuals who suffer from the disorders targeted, so that they see them as complete individuals, not just as patients. The process of deinstitutionalization is already beginning to achieve this for the mentally ill although it may not always seem so. There is evidence that the younger generation are more tolerant of the mentally ill than their parents (Wolff *et al.* 1996*a, b*) and that increased tolerance is associated with knowing someone who is mentally ill.

Wolff's study involved introducing local inhabitants to the residents in a mental health hostel. He found that such exposure resulted in a markedly more positive attitude and more acceptance of these patients. Some of the local inhabitants became involved as visitors to the hostel although this was not the aim of the study. Anything that helps establish the illness as a *part* of the patient's identity rather than *the* identity reduces discrimination and stigma.

Attention to terminology

It is important to address the terminology used in describing disorders. There is a world of difference between saying, "John suffers from Down's syndrome" and saying, "John is a Mongol". Few of us would consider this latter acceptable and learning disability (there it is again) professionals have been enormously successful in forcing these changes through despite accusations of rampant political correctness. Increasingly patients suffering from severe mental illnesses want (quite rightly) to be referred to as 'individuals *suffering from* …' rather than as 'schizophrenics' or 'depressives'. We need to be realistic about this – nobody minds that much being called an asthmatic or hypertensive, it simply does not carry anything like the same sense of pigeonholing or dismissal.

Terms which acquire pejorative overtones need also to be addressed. Learning disabilities practitioners removed terms such as 'idiot' and 'imbecile' (once legitimate, neutral technical designations) from their classification because of their common usage. Doing so does not alter the level of disability of the individual, but it does soften the discourse and allow us to see the individual not just the dramatic and often distorted label. Similarly as 'manic depressive' has become devalued in common use, patients and professionals have welcomed a shift to the term 'bipolar disorder'. Again we need to be realistic – these are not once and for all magic solutions. The new terms may also acquire stigmatizing meanings but they give a breathing space and time to work on educating the population.

Making the individual 'real'

Making the individual real also helps reduce some of the prejudices that are often associated with stigma. Emphasizing, for instance, that there are several ways one can become HIV+ has been important in countering a tendency to dismiss it in some sectors of society as a 'gay plague' that patients brought upon themselves. Distinguishing alcoholism and depression from moral failings have been examples in mental health. Likewise, emphasizing that schizophrenia is not simply the result of excessive drug use or being a Hippie dropout has also helped to remove the stigma surrounding this condition.

'Celebrity endorsement'

Perhaps the most powerful tool in this 'personalization' of mental illnesses is the declaration by well known individuals that they suffer from them. Nothing is as effective in changing public opinion as the witness to their own illness of a popular high-profile figure. It is said that the attitude to the mentally ill was significantly and dramatically improved in 18th century England in response to the very public illness and treatment of the popular King George III. Currently alcohol and drug addictions are regularly acknowledged by high-profile figures, as are eating disorders. These have undoubtedly improved awareness and acceptance of these problems. Depression is increasingly being openly acknowledged (even severe bipolar depression as evidenced by Ted Turner, one of America's richest men) as is Alzheimer's disease by families (e.g. Ronald Reagan, Iris Murdoch). Because of the disabilities associated with it schizophrenia still gets less exposure in this manner although there have recently been very influential Hollywood films portraying schizophrenia in identified individuals in a realistic and sympathetic manner ('Out of Darkness', about a Black singer recovering from schizophrenia with the help of Clozapine, and 'A Beautiful Mind' about the Nobel prize-winning mathematician John Nash who still struggles with his schizophrenia).

Social inclusion: deinstitionalization's second phase

So much space has been devoted here to stigma and discrimination because they are probably the main challenge facing community mental health teams currently. Thirty years ago the challenge was to confront the mental hospitals and enable patients to move out from them. Now the patients are out (and often have never been in for any extensive period); the challenge is to help them overcome the social marginalization that most still experience. It is not enough simply to be out of hospital, we need to make sure our patients are really *in society*. Integration with their peers, suffering the same inconveniences but having the same advantages and opportunities is what they want and what we need to help them achieve.

Social inclusion and integration for most of the mentally ill is both community psychiatry's aim but also, paradoxically, a prerequisite for its success. Unless the life our patients live is dignified and rewarding, we have not finished in our task. If it is not then they will be dissatisfied and reject us and reject our treatments and relapse. The task of the CMHTs described in this book is invariably dual. It involves providing optimal, evidence-based, and increasingly effective treatments to help patients recover. It also involves helping them integrate into their society, with opportunities for friendship and work, which satisfies them without bringing them into such conflict with those around them that the whole unravels.

This commitment to supporting an improved 'quality of life' for our patients (even if it is often not how we would want to live our lives) is not an optional extra. We cannot choose either to focus on effective treatments or on social empowerment. The latter is an integral component of effective treatment for the most severely ill. Without it the treatments will not be sustainable and hence ultimately fail. It is the thesis of this book that the reverse is also true – without effective treatments the social integration of the mentally ill is not feasible. The challenge for CMHTs of all kinds is to attend continually to this balance in their work. It will vary between individual patients and within individual patients over time. There is no fixed answer to it – it is this constant interplay that makes community mental health so dynamic and, ultimately, so rewarding.

CHAPTER 2

Modern multidisciplinary mental health working

Despite doubts about the essential ingredients of community mental health work, multidisciplinary team working is not in question. The movement from institution-based care to the community occurred alongside the development of community mental health teams and the therapeutic community movement. Severe mental illnesses generate a broad range of psychological, behavioural, and social problems. Helping such individuals often requires input in several, if not all, of these areas simultaneously. Trying to do so without adequate understanding and co-ordination between the relevant professionals is at best inefficient and at worst chaotic and confusing for all involved.

> Mental illness places demands on services that no one discipline or agency can meet alone.
>
> (Campbell et al. 1998)

Mental illnesses are characterized by rapid and frequent fluctuations. Clinical and social needs can rarely be predicted and planned for long periods in advance with any certainty (as for instance they may be for some individuals with learning disabilities). In addition different aspects of disability and functioning may vary quite independent of each other. A patient's mental state may deteriorate markedly while their social functioning remains relatively undisturbed (e.g. a paranoid individual's delusions increase in intensity so that he is anxious and distressed but he is able to keep them to himself and continue to attend to his job in a supermarket). Alternatively despite a stable mental state social functioning may decline (e.g. a young man with schizophrenia remains well maintained on clozapine, yet because of a break up with his girlfriend and the subsequent neglect of his hygiene and flat, is faced with possible eviction).

The multidisciplinary community mental health team

The Community Mental Health Team (CMHT) is by definition a multidisciplinary team (increasingly referred to as a 'multi-professional team'). In the UK doctors, nurses and social workers (because of the requirements of the 1959 MHA – see Chapter 1) began to work closely together to organize the care of patients outside the hospital. The first forms of multidisciplinary work were characterized by very clear role divisions with totally separate tasks and responsibilities.

Early descriptions of the doctor–nurse relationship would seem alien to us now – an intensely hierarchical one with the doctor making all the decisions and the nurse following instructions and reporting back on how the patient was doing. Social workers were often only involved where there were issues of housing or finance or when they were needed for compulsory detentions. Often the communication was by letter. Old notes often contain letters from the consultant to the CPN asking them to visit a specific patient and administer depot injections or to an occupational therapist or clinical psychologist asking for an assessment. Although the patient was being offered multidisciplinary input few of us would call this approach a multidisciplinary team.

CMHTs as we recognize them today began to develop when staff from the various disciplines involved in the care of the patient started to meet regularly. These meetings soon evolved beyond the simple process of apportioning tasks. They took on responsibility for jointly reviewing the patient's progress and making joint decisions about treatment plans. *Understanding* the patient's problem also became multifaceted reflecting the multiple components of care.

Role blurring and therapeutic communities

At the same time that CMHTs were rapidly developing, therapeutic communities were a significant feature of mental health practice (Jones 1952). The recognition of social factors in recovery from breakdowns and the central importance of the therapeutic relationship had profoundly altered mental health practice in the 1950s and 1960s (Chapter 1).

This approach recognized that professionals did not just bring their individual professional skills and training to bear in the management of patients. Their personalities were also vital ingredients in the process, as were the more general attitudes and approaches common to the caring professions. Each member of the team brought to the process aspects that were absolutely unique to them, as well as aspects that were shared with several others in the team plus skills and attitudes that could be assumed for all members.

Levels of therapeutic input

◆ Professional training and skills (e.g. medicine, psychology, occupational therapy).
◆ Generic mental health training (e.g. supportive psychotherapy, recognition of psychopathology).
◆ Person skills and temperament (e.g. empathy, compassion, respect for diversity).

Person-skills and temperament

Those of us who choose to work in mental health are not simply a cross-section of society. We are interested in the work for various reasons, both intellectual and personal (often a family experience of mental illness). As a group we are usually fairly identifiable. We are probably more interested in feelings, thoughts, and motivation than in action (perhaps enjoy films and plays slightly more than football). Mental health practitioners are generally 'people people', drawn to interaction with others rather than sitting with computers or repairing cars. These are activities that rely on our ability to understand and enjoy relationships. They prioritize empathy and curiosity. Working with individuals struggling with mental illnesses is no job for rigid conformists. A genuine respect for diversity and different world views is needed. Nor is it a rewarding job for the morally censorious – our patients do sometimes do dreadful things when ill and it is our job to be able to see beyond that to the distressed person.

All of this means that we will tend to be well equipped with the '*person skills*' that all adults need to survive. Empathy, compassion, and being able to understand the other's point of view are essential to adult functioning. Their underdevelopment or absence is a major handicap – most obvious in the extreme examples of psychopathy or autism. Therapeutic Community practice emphasized just how vital these person skills were to effective mental health practice. If staff could not empathize with and support patients then they simply did not recover – despite the provision of the right 'treatments'. At an even more basic level if the staff did not have these skills then patients could not engage with them for treatment.

Role blurring

Therapeutic communities probably over-emphasized the importance of these human characteristics as a counter balance to the prevailing preoccupation with new mental health 'technologies' of the time. However, they remain central to good work and manifest themselves (along with generic mental health skills) most obviously in the concept of '*role blurring*'. Role blurring emphasizes that any member of the team can deliver many of the critical ingredients of good care. The willingness of highly trained staff members to 'stretch' themselves to provide aspects of care that are just outside their job description (but within their personal competence) is viewed as preferable to involving too many individuals with one patient. An obvious example is that the psychiatrist may provide support and encouragement just as much as a nurse may.

While the communality of person-skills has been emphasized a team can also draw on the variation of temperament and individual personality styles within its members. A core of phlegmatic, 'unflappable' staff is needed in any team. Patients need staff who are personally secure and tolerant in order to feel 'contained' and safe. But teams may also have staff who thrive on crises or who can communicate excitement and enthusiasm, and these characteristics can at times be equally valuable. Generic working may often mean that the choice of which key-worker best 'fits' with an individual patient may be driven equally by appropriate professional skills and by individual staff personalities.

Generic mental health training

Not only do different mental health workers find their way into the job for a range of similar reasons there is also a broad overlap in much of their professional training. Most trainings cover the description of the major mental illnesses: their symptoms, course, and treatments. Most also spend time on psychological theories of human functioning and the origins of dysfunction as well as attention to the social factors that exacerbate their development. To a much more variable degree they may also teach the principles and practice of psychotherapies. Currently it is rare for the training of the different professional groups to be shared although the use of common modules is developing (e.g. medical and nursing students may both attend the same seminars on 'breaking bad news' or the care of the dying). The very progressive University of Bangalore in India has had the same first year course for clinical psychologists and psychiatric social workers for over a decade.

As a result it should be rare for any professional to come to a team without knowing the basics of what psychoanalysis is or what antipsychotic drugs are. Clearly their level of familiarity and confidence in using these components of treatment will vary enormously and often be discipline specific. There should, however, be a communality of language and shared concepts.

Professionalism

This communality extends beyond simply a collection of specific skills and knowledge. Of more importance is a shared set of attitudes and values which are conveyed in training. These embody tolerance and acceptance of differing personal priorities, both in ourselves and in our patients. A commitment to advocacy for the disadvantaged and to an inclusive approach to the care of individuals who have for so long been segregated and rejected is required. A common respect for the wishes and priorities of patients, even when we do not share them, is essential if we are to work *with* them rather than *on* them. We often forget just how much of our professional training is devoted to developing appropriate ethics and attitudes. Because we share so much we can become blind to it and forget that untrained staff may need careful induction to the work.

Professional training and skills

The emphasis on role blurring can sometimes be exaggerated and overlook the importance of the team containing a full range of essential skills and competences. Teams are not treatments but vehicles for *delivering* treatments. Unless there are competent individuals in the team who deliver effective treatments then that team is a waste of time – irrespective of how sophisticated its procedures are. This may seem too obvious to warrant mentioning but, as will be clear in subsequent chapters, some teams either lose sight of it or fail to achieve it because of operational issues. The most striking examples are in some Assertive Outreach (AO) teams who consider their job done as long as they engage patients (Chapter 4) or in some Generic CMHTs where territorial and status battles lead to patchy and inconsistent assessment procedures (Chapter 3).

Conflicts over roles and responsibilities within a team only arise and persist if there is some degree of overlap or ambiguity. The unique capacity of medical staff to prescribe does not generate tension on a day to day basis (though it does on a national and interprofessional stage with both clinical psychologists and nurses successfully arguing for a change in legislation). Few competencies or skills are, however, purely restricted to one professional group. Most professions working in the CMHT have an identified 'lead' in some procedures but overlap with other professions in others and no involvement at all in still others. Figure 2.1 is an attempt to map the distributions and overlap of these expertises in a US rehabilitation service. The distribution of leadership expertise is intriguing. The picture is, in reality, even more complicated. The 'average' professional distributions in Fig. 2.1 will be further influenced by levels of training and experience of individual staff members.

There is a tension between a professional focus and generic working that has to be worked out in all CMHTs. It would be misleading to suggest there is any 'one-off' answer to this question. It will depend on the range of problems dealt with, the composition of the team, the complexity and duration of treatments and even on such basic issues as population density. It is in Generic CMHTs and Early Intervention Teams where these controversies are currently most intense. CMHTs have grappled with them longest. Unacknowledged rivalries based on professional status are the commonest cause of a local failure of resolution. Status rivalries are nothing to be ashamed about – they are part of the human condition. What can make them pernicious in mental health is that our democratic and inclusive traditions can lead us to pretend they are not there. If we have learnt anything from psychotherapy it is that conflicts need to be acknowledged and explored if they are going to be resolved. It may be enough that we understand each other's position on such matters for the team to work well, even if there is not full agreement.

Team functioning

The essence of a team is that a varied group of individuals regularly meet face-to-face. Within CMHTs this means meeting *at least* once a week. How such meetings are configured will depend very much on the nature of the team and their individual purpose. Some teams will have several meetings of different types for different reasons (e.g. an AO team may have daily handovers and a weekly in-depth review meeting). Not only will the format of the meetings vary but their composition may do so (e.g. the medics may not be present at the shift handover in a Home Treatment/Crisis Resolution team). However there will always be 'a team meeting' where all the team are present and which is usually understood by those present as 'the team meeting'.

Areas of Expertise	Psychiatrist	Psychologist	Social Worker	Nurse	Occupational Therapist	Rehabilitation Therapist	Case Manager	Consumer Team Member	Family Advocate	Employment Specialist	Job Coach
Diagnosis	4	3	1	1	0	1	1	0	1	1	0
Monitoring psychopathology	4	3	1	3	1	1	2	1	0	2	2
Crisis intervention	4	4	2	4	0	0	4	2	1	2	0
Engagement in treatment	2	2	2	2	1	1	4	4	2	4	4
Motivational interviewing	1	3	2	0	2	2	1	3	0	4	2
Functional assessment	1	4	2	0	4	0	1	1	0	3	2
Psychopharmacology	4	2	0	2	0	0	1	2	1	2	1
Family psychoeducation	2	3	4	1	0	0	1	1	3	0	0
Patient psychoeducation	3	4	1	3	1	0	1	2	1	0	0
Skills training	1	4	1	1	2	0	2	1	0	2	3
Cognitive-behavioral therapy	2	4	1	0	0	1	0	0	0	0	0
Supported employment	0	4	2	0	2	1	1	1	0	4	4
Assertive Community Treatment	2	1	3	2	2	0	4	4	1	1	1
Team leadership	2	2	2	2	0	0	0	0	0	0	0
Program development	2	2	2	1	1	0	0	0	0	1	0
Cultural competence	1	2	2	2	1	0	2	4	4	0	0

4 = Highest expectations
0 = Lowest expectations

Fig. 2.1 Expected expertise in psychiatric rehabilitation of team members from different disciplines (Adapted from Liberman et al. 2001)

Without such a meeting teams are usually doomed and certainly where senior staff routinely absent themselves from the meetings teams rarely flourish (Liberman *et al.* 2001).

Teams are also important for staff. It is not simply to cover the range of skills for effective input to patients and families but to provide a working environment that is rewarding and sustains excellence. Figure 2.2 is an attempt to overview these different roles that team-working may fulfil in mental health. Professional support and development are legitimate requirements in a service, nothing to be ashamed of. If the service structure does not offer support and educational and promotion opportunities then it will not attract or retain good staff and ultimately the patients will be the losers. Often very radical and innovative services have ignored the sustainability for staff of their approach (Wright *et al.* 2000).

Burnout

Burnout has become a topic of increasing importance in mental health services. The emotional demands of our work, dealing daily with human distress and misfortune, have been compounded by a critical and demanding society that no longer takes our goodwill on trust. Research studies on burnout are often quite confusing and contradictory (Onyett *et al.* 1997) but there is a clear consensus that job satisfaction and burnout vary enormously in the same job between different settings. Team membership, and in particular being a member of a team which is well led and clearly focused, seems to be a powerful protector against premature burnout. At its most basic we can remind each other that we are doing good work even if the patient and family do not appreciate it.

Case Example

Frank came to the AO team after a stormy 10-year history of repeated compulsory admissions for his schizophrenia. He lived alone in a council flat that was eccentrically and strikingly decorated when he was well but became a serious health hazard with rotting food and electric fires left on when he became ill. Relapses were severe with gross disorganization and neglect and frequently associated with exploitation and even assault from the local community. He was a very intelligent man with an interest in reading and philosophy and a formidable debater (usually about not wanting medication).

Over four years of contact 3–4 times a week he has continued with medication and only had two brief voluntary admissions of a couple of weeks each. He has made contact with his adult son and can get to the library. However he adamantly refuses to do anything else. He has had to go back to depot medication and will only see his key-worker every one or two weeks. He continues to give his key-worker a hard time at every visit. Not surprisingly his key-worker has become demoralized 'am I really doing anything? All I'm doing is giving him his depot, he might as well be with his CMHT'.

The team, however, are able to reflect back just how much better things are than the nightmare for everyone before he settled. A discussion ensued about how we cope with stable but 'unrewarding' (or as GPs call them 'heartsink') patients and some plans about transferring key-worker responsibility at sensible intervals was proposed. Alan felt much better about himself – and just as important better about his work with Frank.

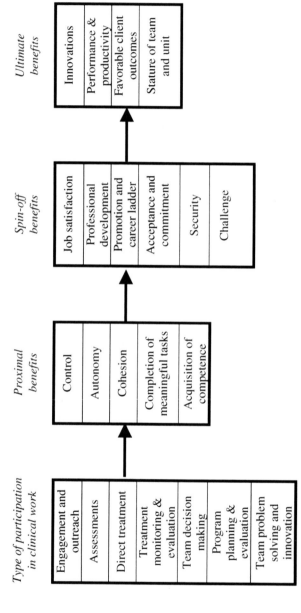

Fig. 2.2 Conceptual map of participatory teamwork and its benefits (Adapted from Liberman *et al.* 2001)

Team dynamics

So far the benefits of working as a team have been stressed. There are, however, down-sides. It is undeniable that personality clashes and disagreements are common in any team. There are three main contributors to conflict in CMHTs.

Causes of conflict in CMHTs

- ◆ Professional differences.
- ◆ Personality differences.
- ◆ Projection and splitting.

Professional differences

Teams are constituted *because* the members differ and can bring different perspectives and contributions. In CMHTs these differences reflect professional roles and responsibilities which have considerable overlap. As mentioned above, it is rarely black and white who should do what in a team. Where it is there is little scope for conflict or 'dynamics'. Because of the role-blurring and overlap in CMHTs, however, there is a constant need for clarity and discussion about who is doing what and why they are doing it.

It is best if there is a clear team operational policy that addresses the issues of profession-specific responsibilities. This will not solve the whole problem. A CMHT has to be flexible and rapidly responsive to changing needs in its patients. The obvious role of one team member today may not be so appropriate tomorrow – somebody else's skills may be right or the relative importance of differing inputs may change because of an increased urgency. There is not always a right answer in these situations so judgement and mutual respect are of great importance.

A very chaotic young mother had been cared for by the team for just over two years. Her severe mood swings had been contained, if not controlled. She was receiving a lowdose depot from the CPN who had supported and encouraged her to persist with treatment and resist overdosing and acting out. As a consequence of her improved stability she had been encouraged by the CPN and the whole team to get psychotherapeutic help with earlier abuse which still haunted her. She had been seeing the team psychologist weekly for 3–4 months.

Initially things had gone very well and everyone was delighted by her progress. However in the last few weeks she had become distraught and taken two quite risky overdoses (one alone with a young child in the house). The psychologist believed the treatment was at last getting somewhere and the current crises were an essential, though temporary and distressing, phase and that the treatment should continue uninterrupted. The CPN also felt that the treatment was right for the patient but that the risks were too great. She had stepped up her contact with the patient but believed that things would get impossible if the psychotherapy was not halted or at least slowed down for a time.

Here two experienced colleagues have come to different conclusions about management based on differing training and differing experiences. Both positions reflect complex clinical judgements and neither can be 'proved right'. The team will have to recognize a legitimate professional difference of opinion. It must come to a balanced pragmatic decision which benefits the patient and, hopefully, does not leave either professional feeling criticized or humiliated.

Personality differences

Mental health work is stressful and we cannot be saints all the time. A range of personalities strengthens a team – using one's own personality is a recognized aspect of practice. Occupational therapy has paid particular attention to this and 'the use of the self' in treatment is a strength in their training (Willson 1987). Faced with a complex approach to a patient's problem some staff will be tolerant (perhaps favouring a slower supportive approach), others impatient, favouring grasping the nettle and confrontation. Obviously the choice of the terms 'tolerant' and 'impatient' seems moralistic and the same dilemma could be presented using terms like 'diffident' and 'confident' etc. The issues may be tiny or momentous but wherever judgement is being exercised this will be coloured by personality and experience. It is not a sensible approach to try and eradicate this dimension in decision making. It needs to be recognized and addressed if it is distorting decision outcomes.

Dominant personalities

Strong personalities can enrich a team but they can also pose serious problems. If team members consistently respond in a manner that really does not benefit the patient (e.g. too abrasive, or even too accepting and sensitive) then this needs to be taken up with them in supervision. People cannot easily change their personalities. However, being aware of their natural tendencies can help them compensate for them and, indeed, exploit them more successfully.

A more serious problem arises when the personality of a team member affects other staff and may interfere with smooth working. The commonest problem is the dominant individual with strong opinions who inhibits discussion and consideration of issues. Pedantic or intensely focused staff can also severely disrupt effective functioning. If they have preoccupations about aspects of treatment about which they are very knowledgeable and strong advocates, but remain ignorant of the range of alternative opinions or approaches, their contributions can be very restricting. Resentment (and even envy) can be generated by such people. They are not real *'team players'* and can easily become isolated and scapegoated. Resolving these sorts of problems often needs a team acknowledgement and discussion of the issue in addition to individual supervision.

Projection and splitting

All teams have to deal with professional rivalries and personality difficulties – it is not restricted to CMHTs. Mental health services, however, have an extra dimension to problems in team working, which comes from their patients. Projection and splitting are the two processes that psychoanalysts have described which most affect the functioning of mental health teams (Jones 1952; Main 1946; Sandler *et al.* 1992). Essentially these are unconscious processes within the patient which affect how they relate emotionally to the staff who are treating them. They reflect problems they have had in relationships earlier in their lives and which are still troubling them. In effect they involve the staff around them to re-enact these earlier conflicts in a repetitive and pathological manner. If staff are not aware of what is going on they can very easily be drawn into the process.

Projection

A simple example is of a patient who has been neglected or denigrated as a child. They have grown up insecure about whether anyone can really like or respect them. Consequently they desperately need to believe that their new nurse is not like everyone else they have met in the past. The patient is convinced that any normal person will soon tire of them and reject them – only a 'perfect' individual could know them as they really are and yet not abandon them. They may deal with this by projecting on to the new nurse the qualities of a perfect person 'idealizing' them. This process can be very powerful and subtly the nurse comes to believe that they are 'absolutely right' for this patient, and becomes over-involved and loses perspective. There are many examples of patients projecting qualities on to staff that we then begin to believe or act on – and not always pleasant ones.

Splitting

Projection is even more damaging in teams because it so often leads to splitting. It is particularly common in patients who have grown up without the experience of successful compromise and mutual respect within a family. They may have only been able to survive in angry and conflict-ridden situations in the past by forming a strong alliance with one parent against the other in the dispute. This internal conflict is projected onto different team members.

> To the doctor: 'You understand me but the nurses are simply unable to see how it has been. They just ignore me.'
> To the nurses: 'My problems are really severe and complex. It takes someone like Dr Jones to understand them. He's helping but you're making it worse.'

In successful splitting the doctors and nurses start to become annoyed with each other seeing each other through the patients' eyes. The result is tension in the team and everybody working against one another. Splitting is often not so explicit – behaviour is a more potent force than words. This behaviour can be dramatic (e.g. a team can be thrown into discord by patients who repeatedly cut and overdose) or insidious (e.g. a steady gratifying response to the input from some staff and stubborn resistance to that from others). The remarkable feature of splitting is that we genuinely begin to feel and believe the attributes, both good and bad, projected onto us (often called 'projective identification' in psychoanalytic circles).

These are very powerful forces and in the past mental health staff received extensive psychodynamic training in understanding and spotting them. Therapeutic communities devoted a significant part of the working week to staff groups to keep a check on these dynamics and make sure that staff were all pulling in the same direction. Psychodynamic thinking has fallen somewhat out of fashion and currently staff have little training in this area or time or support dedicated to it.

Dealing with team dynamics

Teams deal with these dynamic issues in a number of ways. It used to be popular to have an hour a week or fortnight when the team discussed its own functioning with or without a facilitator. Discussion could develop out of current patient issues or just deal with team tensions. This can be very helpful but needs to be carefully handled – much will depend on the facilitator if one is used. Many teams have found using a facilitator feels too artificial, especially when the discussion is pitched at the interface between a current management issue and team responses. A facilitator who really does not understand the clinical issues can be a serious distraction.

Distinguishing professional from therapeutic relationships

There are basic rules to be observed. The commonest mistake is to use the same approach that one uses in therapy with patients. This is not appropriate – colleagues are colleagues, they are not patients. They need to feel safe and in control of what information they divulge (for instance if a personal problem is affecting how they are currently coping at work). Often information that is not appropriate to the team to know will be known to the team leader only, and the leader may have to intervene to maintain boundaries. This can be even more important where young staff are at risk of exposing themselves in ways they may later regret.

Although formal team dynamic sessions are now rare many teams ensure that they have a culture where emotional responses can be explored as part of their routine work. Often this will be in reviews of difficult patients. Much depends on the skill of the team leader to ensure an open and safe culture in the team – staff must not be penalized for expressing anxiety and uncertainty. Similarly teams have to learn to contain disagreement without bullying or recourse to insults. The voices of quiet or diffident staff need equal airing in the team.

Dynamics can be addressed in away-days (see 'Team size'). If time is not set aside apart from away-days then the approach needs to be fairly formal such as in a SWOT (Strengths, Weaknesses, Opportunities, Threats) analysis. Only when teams are safe with disclosure and able to deal with it on a regular basis is a very personal approach profitable. If it is being reserved for a team day then almost by definition this is not the case. Experiences with psychodynamic facilitators on team days is rarely rewarding.

Team size

The effectiveness of a team is limited by the ability of the members to know each other well and to meet regularly face-to-face. As teams get larger, adding more and more skills, the losses in terms of familiarity and difficulties in meeting may begin to outweigh the advantages. The exact upper limit of the team is dependent on several factors. Less acute teams can function with larger numbers as the decision-making processes are not so time constrained. When the proportion of part-time staff in a team increases the overall optimal size reduces because of information transfer problems. Teams of about 10–12 individuals seem optimal for providing a sufficient range of skills but ensuring familiarity. There are only so many combinations any of us can keep in our head. Current CMHTs are often up to 14–16 staff and the recommendations for Home Treatment/Crisis Resolution teams and Early Intervention Service (EIS) teams are much above this (20+). These larger teams work on shift systems where the shift operates essentially as a sub-team.

Teams of less than about 6 full time staff have a history of not surviving. One has to anticipate that with annual leave, various training obligations and sickness the average staff member is only present 3 weeks out of 4. In addition, most staff prefer not to be the only representative of their discipline on the team (the only social worker, the only doctor etc.). As discussed above the team needs to provide important professional development support for staff and this generally requires a critical mass.

Team leadership

Different types of teams require different types of leadership and this is addressed in the subsequent chapters. Strong leadership is routinely identified as a quality of successful teams, though often without describing or defining exactly what this quality is. It is certainly a complex concept, ranging from a rather nebulous role of inspiring and infusing a team with a sense of direction, through to a more concrete role directing individual team members in quite explicit detail. Where teams are mainly composed of professional staff a 'micro-management' approach from the team leader is neither warranted nor usually successful. In mental health teams the leader's role is one of harnessing the skills of the team and monitoring (and occasionally correcting) the direction of travel with a gentle touch on the tiller.

Leadership and management

Leadership and managerial roles can be invested in the same individual or kept separate. A managerial role implies a tighter, day-to-day control of the team. Usually this will involve a range of tasks including scheduling shifts and annual leave, monitoring activity returns and sickness, prompting continuing professional development, audit and appraisal. These are essential tasks to maintain the effectiveness of the team and skills and performance of individual members. Not surprisingly team managers often acquire a leadership role.

Where the two roles are separate it is vital that their relationship is a close one and one that is well defined and understood by all the team. No relationship is more prone to the 'splitting' described above than that between team leader and manager. Leaders can, thoughtlessly, allow the manager to be responsible for all the difficult, day to day decisions, standing aloof from them and becoming the 'good guy'. This is never sensible. Care must be taken to identify both roles with the decisions that have to be taken – even though their executive function may differ in the process.

Management and supervision

Where team managers also carry a significant responsibility for professional supervision (often the case where the manager is a senior nurse and several of the team are nurses) this can be very effective but is also a tricky balance. Arranging for staff support independent of direct managerial accountability is one solution. For instance in the Wandsworth ACT team (Burns and Firn 2002a) the team manager is a nurse and provides clinical supervision to all the non-medical staff on the team (nursing, OT, and Social work). A nurse practitioner on the team conducts a staff support/development group within the team. In this meeting (which has an explicit fire-wall between it and the management function) professional and personal doubts and difficulties within the team can be expressed and worked with. This approach reflects the 'generic' approach to key-working within the AO team. Individual staff can seek more specialized supervision and professional advice within their discipline outside the team (e.g. the social worker with a senior social worker, the OT with a senior OT).

Who is on the team?

Leadership, management, support, and supervision are four vital components of a successful team. As will be obvious from this brief introduction there is more than one way to distribute and configure them in a team. Their disposition and combinations will depend primarily on a team's characteristics, its obligations, and tasks. The individuals on the team, however, will also influence it very powerfully. Individual strengths and skills cannot, and should not, be ignored. For instance the role of the nurse practitioner in the staff support group in the Wandsworth ACT team described above was only possible because one of the staff was highly skilled and this, along with his input to teaching, resulted in his promotion to nurse practitioner. There was no practitioner post established in the team so without this unique individual this particular configuration could not have been considered. As it was it worked very well, but since his departure alternatives have had to be found.

Diversity

Balancing diversity with shared skills and attributes is a never-ending issue in mental health teams. Teams must share enough in their understanding of their patients' problems and a core vision of how best to help them if they are to pull together in any meaningful manner. Within this framework diversity in team members is a strength. Diversity is both professional and personal. The professional diversity needs to cover the required treatments and skills (Fig. 2.1). In addition a range of temperaments supports therapeutic relationships with the varied personalities and needs of individual patients.

Ethnic variety

It is desirable that a team reflects the community it serves. This is particularly important in areas with sizeable minority ethnic populations. Ethnic matching has been proposed by some workers but is now rarely viewed as an important objective – even if it were feasible. What matters is that the team itself is sufficiently similar to those it serves. That way patients can have confidence that the staff have some real understanding of their life experiences. Young black men will generally have experienced considerable ethnic stereotyping and discrimination and need to feel that staff understand the origins and nature of their distrust of authorities. Similarly Asian women need to feel reassured that their particular perspective, often incorporating a profound sense of submission and dependence based on traditional gender roles, will be understood, and that clinical advice and judgements will not all reflect an exclusively white middle-class standpoint.

This diversity is good for patients but also good for the team members who benefit from having their assessments enriched by having more than one take on things. A broad and tolerant approach, which recognizes and respects the varied cultures patients are drawn from, may promote a more accurate understanding of their problems. It will invariably enrich decision making about prioritising differing interventions. Community mental health is increasingly confronted by complex ethical challenges, often balancing needs for care against individual autonomy and independence. These ethical decisions cannot be disengaged from the patient's and their family's culture. Ethnic diversity in the team does not necessarily mean that if the patient is Asian then the decision will be decided by an Asian member of staff (though obviously their insights are invaluable). Indeed minority ethnic staff often complain about the unrealistic expectations that can be placed on them

> 'Okay Costas, you must be able to help Mrs Liakos disengage from Greg. They really are complicated and intense these Greek families!'

What it does mean is that the team never loses sight of the cultural relativism of so many of our decisions, not just those involving ethnic minorities.

Procedures and paperwork

Getting the balance right between a robust and reliable recording system without overloading the service with bureaucracy is a real challenge in modern mental health care. There is currently a seemingly inexorable pressure from above to capture all aspects of our work in predesigned forms. Ever since the Ritchie enquiry into the homicide by

Christopher Clunis (Ritchie 1994) there has been a preoccupation with the failure of service staff to note or pass on essential information that could influence subsequent decisions. This is a legitimate concern – had what was known about Clunis been easily available to subsequent duty doctors when he was assessed then the risk he posed might have been recognized and different clinical decisions made. A level of consistency about the recording of care and clinical decisions is now required that goes well beyond traditional practices of simply 'keeping good notes'.

Reviews

SMI patients rapidly acquire voluminous case notes. Information is hard to find and previous decisions get overlooked and lost. Regular, structured reviews of care are essential both to ensure that there is an up to date and accessible summary of the current clinical approach and also to make sure that clinical care does not drift. There is a real risk that we become so familiar with their patients over time that we fail to notice important clinical changes that ought to prompt a change in treatment plan (Wooff et al. 1988). Structuring the clinical review is one way of dealing with this. Many teams use validated assessment tools such as the Brief Psychiatric Rating Scale (BPRS, Overall and Gorham 1962) or the Beck Depression scale (Beck et al. 1961) to strengthen the review. In the UK and Australia Health of the Nation Outcome Scale (HoNOS, Wing et al. 1999) has been introduced as a repeat measure of clinical and social function specifically to be used at reviews.

The Care Programme Approach

It was a series of tragedies that accelerated the Care Programme Approach (CPA) (Department of Health 1990) in the UK. In many other countries the recording of care has always been considerably better, not least because it is the base for billing. Although there was considerable resistance in the UK to the introduction of the CPA most professionals have come to value it as an essential minimum of recording. The CPA requires that each patient in the secondary services who needs complex or ongoing care should have an identified 'keyworker' and a formal care plan in the notes. The keyworker (now referred to as 'care co-ordinator') is responsible for drawing up and reviewing the care plan. The care plan must, as a minimum, include the patient's identified needs and the interventions proposed to meet these listed. It must indicate who is responsible for meeting these needs (often the key-worker, but not always) and it must be signed by the keyworker and have a date for review noted.

Enhanced and standard tiers

The above are the absolute basics for so-called 'enhanced CPA' – an infuriating aspect of this form of central bureaucracy is that the terms keep changing. For 'standard' CPA (where there is only a simple single discipline intervention, often short term) then special forms are generally no longer required. There have been a series of directives about the CPA. Virtually all of these (e.g. that the patient, and where possible carer, are fully involved and receive copies of the plan, that special attention to issues such as dual diagnosis and cultural factors receive adequate attention) are very sensible. The problem is institutionalizing them and designing forms that include all of them even when they are obviously irrelevant to specific patients.

The result is that CPA tends to work well where there has been significant local clinical involvement in the design of the forms. Left to senior managers or committees the forms invariably become longer and longer (12 pages in one London Trust). Paperwork is meant to support good clinical practice and not impede it and a strong stand has to be taken to keep CPA documents useable. The form shown in Fig. 2.3 is that used in the adult directorate of the SW London and St George's MH Trust. We set an absolute limit that it should be kept to one A4 side. This required rigor as everyone involved in its development had some pet issue that (often for very understandable reasons) they wanted recorded.

Balancing therapy and bureaucracy

While increased richness of data can improve audit and clinical governance it can obscure the information transfer that is the primary purpose of the CPA. If the crucial message about a patient's vulnerability and need for consistent daily monitoring of medication compliance is lost in a wealth of information about housing and family contact numbers the battle may be lost. This has been most obvious in the thinking around risk assessment (see below). After a rather panicky response which involved the adoption of long, unvalidated tick box questionnaires of risk factors by many services, there has been a reversal to a more contextualized risk assessment. In these the professional is prompted about areas to cover but writes down the important issues only.

Similarly if the paperwork is too prescriptive it undermines the normal professional position of continually making decisions for which we are personally, professionally responsible. Professionals are expected always to check the situation and make sure they are content with what they are doing with a patient. We do not do something simply because we are instructed to, no matter how senior the instruction or the confidence and detail of a written directive. Over-prescriptive paperwork can induce a state of unthinking obedience in professional staff that is in nobody's interest.

There remain doubts about many aspects of the implementation of the CPA (such as the use of clumsy and misleading terms like 'needs'). However it is still the basis of the review process in most teams in the UK and reflects closely that which is used in most developed countries. The form in Fig. 2.3, while far from perfect, is brief and focused. It has proved itself useable in day to day practice.

Contingency planning and risk assessment

The CPA document in Fig. 2.3 clearly indicates that risk should be assessed for every patient. For most patients this is simply a brief check of whether there is either a

ENHANCED CPA REVIEW

Patient's name:	**CMHT:**
Address:	**Phone:**
	New patient: YES/NO
Phone:	**If NO, date of review: ....**
Date of birth:	**Diagnosis:**
GP:	1.. F __ __ . __
Phone:	2.. F __ __ . __

You must consider the following:

1) Mental health, including indicators of relapse;
2) Physical health;
3) Medication;
4) Daytime activity;
5) Personal care / living skills;
6) Carers, family, children and social network;

7) Forensic history; 8) Alcohol or substance misuse;
9) Cultural factors; 10) Housing/finances/legal issues; and
a) make sure a **risk assessment** is done;
b) include: **i) a crisis plan;   ii) a contingency plan**
i.e. what should be done if part of the careplan can't be
be provided(e.g. the care co-ordinator is on leave or ill)

Assessed needs or problem	Intervention	Resp.of

Professionals involved in care: Dr.   Psychologist   CPN   OT   SW   Ward Nurse   ACT   Support Worker Other

Present at planning meeting: Dr.   Psychologist   CPN   OT   SW   Ward Nurse   ACT   Support Worker Other

Plan discussed with the   YES/NO   Copy given to patient?   YES/NO   Copy sent to GP?   **YES/NO**

Care co-ordinator (print):   **Phone**

Care co-ordinator (signature):   ....   **Date of next review: ....**

Job title: **Patient's signature: ....**

Care management? **YES/NO**	Risk history completed? **YES/NO**
On Supervised Discharge? **YES/NO**	Relapse + risk plan required? **YES/NO**

Fig. 2.3 Enhanced care plan (SW London and St George's Mental Health Trust)

history or current evidence of risk any of the following areas:

- Harm to self (e.g. overdosing, reckless behaviour in a disinhibited state).
- Aggression or violence (e.g. threats, hostility or even aggression).
- Severe self-neglect (e.g. not eating, leaving the cooker on).
- Exploitation (e.g. being threatened by local drug dealers).
- Risk to children (rare but important).

For most patients there will be no significant history or current risk. For these no more needs to be done other than to confirm with a tick on the Care Plan that the assessment has been conducted and that no relapse and risk plan is required. If, however, there is evidence of risk then a relapse plan (Fig. 2.4) and risk history (Fig. 2.5) should be completed and distributed to the relevant agencies (i.e. GP, A&E, social services).

Such review forms need to be locally adapted and probably regularly reviewed to make sure that they reflect current practice. Vigilance to resist their expansion will be needed at each of these reviews.

Assessments

There have been several attempts to devise assessment forms for differing teams. One driver for these forms comes from a desire to formalize the primary care/secondary care threshold – to establish criteria and guidelines for referral. Another driver is from social services' experience of having to use junior and inexperienced staff to conduct high volumes of brief assessments in the context of strict accountability. Having a template for the interview gives a sense of security that all the important issues will be covered. It also may mean that experience will build up over time about the relevant criteria for transfer between one service and another.

Structured referral forms

The approach advanced in this book is based on a recognition of the endless variety of presentations of mental health problems and the value of their assessment by well trained staff. In both generic CMHTs and Crisis Resolution/Home Treatment teams (Chapters 3 and 6) it is usual practice to restrict assessments to medical or highly experienced non-medical professionals. In crisis teams (where a preliminary screen may be conducted by a relatively junior team member over the phone) the structured data collection can serve the same purposes as those outlined for social services (see Chapter 6). In the AO and EIS teams assessments are more leisurely and allow for supervision and review within the team in cases of uncertainty. It is debatable if anything is to be gained in terms of increased rigor or quality of assessment in such teams by using structured assessment forms.

CONFIDENTIAL: RELAPSE AND RISK MANAGEMENT PLAN

Name:

Categories of Risk Identified:

Aggression and violence	YES/NO	Severe self-neglect	YES/NO
Exploitation (self or others)	YES/NO	Risk to children & young adults	YES/NO
Suicide and self-harm	YES/NO	Other (please specify)	

Current factors which suggest there is significant apparent risk:
(For example: alcohol or substance misuse; specific threats; suicidal ideation; violent fantasies; anger; suspiciousness; persecutory beliefs; paranoid feelings or ideas about particular people)

Clear statement of anticipated risk(s):
(Who is at risk; how immediate is that risk; how severe; how ongoing)

Action Plan:
(Including names of people responsible for each action and steps to be taken if plan breaks down)

Date Completed: xx/xx/xx   **Review date:**   xx/xx/xx

This risk assessment may contain confidential and/or sensitive information provided by third parties. Such information should not be disclosed to the patient without prior consultation with the informant

SW London and St George's Mental Health Trust

Fig. 2.4 Relapse plan

Early feedback from users of NHS Direct and also some local crisis lines indicates that callers dislike highly structured questioning. They want to tell their story and explain their problems and they find too many questions intrusive and off-putting. Skill and tact are required in getting this balance right. We need the information, but not at the cost of alienating those who need the service.

Where such forms do help is in the collection of statistics for reporting on the team's activity and for developing a more accurate understanding within the team of its practice. The EIS assessment form presented in Chapter 5 is an example of a structured

RISK ASSESSMENT DOCUMENTATION

Client's Name:

RISK HISTORY

Give details of any risk behaviour shown by the patient (actual or threatened). Each entry must be signed and dated
(E.g. previous violence; weapons used; impulsivity; self-harm; non-compliance; disengagement from services; convictions; potentially seriously harmful acts)

SW London and St George's Mental Health Trust

Fig. 2.5 Risk history

assessment completed at the face-to-face interview which is used in this way. For teams with high referral and assessment rates it is unclear whether the effort expended in such form-filling is productive or not.

Communication

Structured discharge summaries and letters to GPs are popular with many services so that there is no delay in communication. These supplement, but do not substitute for, the more considered letters that should accompany changes in treatment or transfers. Usually they only contain details of current medication and the date of the follow-up appointment. Their advantage is their brevity and simplicity. Nothing at all is gained by making them more complex. Redundant material is not just a waste but risks obscuring important communications. We are all aware of the different level of attention we pay to circulars as opposed to personal letters which come through our letter boxes.

Mental health professionals have gained confidence over the last two decades in allowing patients access to their notes (Kosky and Burns 1995). Not only have we found that generally it does no harm but it is a positive step in the move to more equal partnership with patients exercising more responsibility for their treatment. Adequate attention has to be paid to protection of third party information. The current policy of sending copies of GP letters to patients can only be to the good as long as common sense is used. Some patients are very sensitive about their family knowing of their contact with us and do not want communication home. Others may not be able to read and regularly ask neighbours (or their key-worker) to read letters for them. Consideration has to be given in such exceptional circumstances but otherwise keeping the patient in the communication loop is overwhelmingly positive.

Governance and audit

A very patient-centred approach often makes it difficult to be aware of the overall performance of a team. We are so concerned to tailor the care we provide for each unique individual that it is very easy to lose sight of whether or not we are delivering the effective and evidence-based treatments that are available to all who need them. It is to ensure that what happens on a day to day basis approaches what we know to be best practice that audit and clinical governance are so essential. Whenever the practice of mental health care is audited it is found to be well below agreed aspirations (Lehman and Steinwachs 1998).

Clinical governance is the system set up to monitor practice and control for both the content of the care (i.e. which treatments are offered) and also to get feedback on the quality of those treatments. A basic first step in clinical governance is to collect accurate and reliable data on what is going on. This includes simple contact data but also information on complex interventions and, more ambitiously, patient and carer feedback on their experience and level of satisfaction with the care offered. These are difficult issues – assessing the quality of an intervention or satisfaction with services are not amenable to simple questionnaires. However, they are often measured in just that way despite the methodological complications of measuring quality in mental health care (James and Burns 2002).

Clinical governance systems are of varying complexity and development in different services. An absolute minimum is that services should be able to report routinely and easily how many patients they have assessed in the last year and how many patients they currently have on their books. This may seem ridiculously basic but, remarkably, it is often not available. The different types of forms surveyed in this chapter can also contribute to improving this level of information so that the diagnoses, age, gender, and ethnic mix of assessments and caseload can be monitored to check equality of access. Times between referral and assessment, between discharge and follow up and the relevant letters to the GP can also give simple indications of quality and accessibility.

Care pathways

Care pathways are attracting a lot of interest in medicine although as yet there are no widely accepted examples within mental health. Care pathways are a means of formally marrying routine clinical procedures to evidence-based guidelines for best practice. They are generally referred to as 'Integrated care pathways' (ICPs), defined thus:

> Integrated care pathways are structured multidisciplinary care plans which detail essential steps in the care of patients with a specific clinical problem.

> (Campbell *et al.* 1998)

They have been most developed in surgery or in areas of technologically sophisticated medicine where the interventions are discrete and unequivocal. They can obviously only be used when there is an evidence base for the intervention.

The most likely format for their use in mental health is as a checklist of evidence-based components of the care package. This would be completed at major transition points in the patient's care (of their 'pathway' through the care process) such as referral, admission or discharge, and possibly eventually at routine CPA reviews.

Features of care pathways

- ◆ Structured.
- ◆ Multidisciplinary.
- ◆ Records reasons for departure from guidelines.

Fig. 2.6 shows part of a care pathway for the discharge of patients after cardiac catheterization. As can be seen it has broken the process down into very clearly defined, discrete interventions – it is highly *structured*. One part is for the nursing staff to complete and another for the medical staff – it is *multidisciplinary*. In mental health it could quite easily include other crucial disciplines such as social work and psychology or occupational therapy – particularly where their inputs are sufficiently discrete and defined. Lastly (and perhaps most importantly, given the resistance of many mental health professionals to prescriptive guidelines) it *records variation, alternative actions, and the reasons for them* (Table 2.1).

As well as a quality assurance tool the care pathway is a learning tool. It encourages knowledge of the evidence base but also respects the need for clinical decisions and asks for these to be recorded. The audit (and indeed research potential) of this information must be obvious. Despite this integrated care pathways have their detractors (Campbell *et al.* 1998).

The most obvious problem in mental health is the absence of accepted disorder-specific guidelines. There are some local and national pharmacotherapy algorithms (such as the National Institute for Clinical Excellence (NICE) guidance in schizophrenia) but these are not sufficiently detailed to form the basis of a care pathway. East Anglia Mental Health Trust has made progress on a schizophrenia ICP which includes 18 components, the main ones of which are shown in Table 2.2. Each of the 18 components has one or several detailed steps that are required. Time will tell if this approach is successfully applicable within CMHT practice or not.

Audit in care pathways

Where services have agreed standards these can be audited as part of clinical governance. For instance time to assessment in CMHTs (Chapter 3) or the provision of

---

Medical Assessment Pre-Discharge

Date: ___ / ___ / ___

Clinical findings: _____

_____

_____

_____

Results of investigations (if required)

FBC: _____

CXR: _____

ECHO: _____

_____

_____

_____

Other: _____

DISCHARGED Y ❑   N ❑   Date of discharge ___ / ___ / ___

If No, document reason and information given to family:

Medication:

Doctor's Signature: _____

PRE-DISCHARGE ASSESSMENT DATE ___ / ___ / ___		
Nurses to complete	Variance, Reason & Action taken	Signed
Patient taking and tolerating fluids and solids ❑		
If child discharged on day of cath wound checked ❑		
No haematoma/bleeding ❑		
Dressing removed day after catheter by nurse or parent ❑		
Limbs well perfused - warm, pink, pulses present ❑		
4 hourly obs within acceptable range ❑		
Abonormalities reported to Dr _____		
IVT and monitoring discontinued ❑		
All requested investigations carried out ❑		

DISCHARGE INFORMATION		
Discharged on ___ / ___ / ___		
Give post catheter advice sheet to parents ❑		
Give TTO and drug advice sheet to parents ❑		
Ensure patient/family's understanding of the above ❑		
Address any other concerns that family may have ❑		
Health visitor/school nurse referral via HISS ❑		
OPA Date given __/__/__ (See Dr's info to ward staff)		

This record is for Cardiac Catheterisation only. If a child remains an outpatient for any reason, a full clinical assessment must be carried out and a care plan written.

Fig. 2.6 Cardiac catheterization care pathway: pre-discharge checklist

Table 2.1 Integrated care pathways: pros and cons

Proponents of ICPs say that they:

- Facilitate the introduction of research-based evidence into local protocols.
- Result in more complete and accessible data collection for audit.
- Encourage multidisciplinary communication and care planning.
- Promote more patient-focused care by letting the patient see what is planned.
- Enable staff to learn quickly the key interventions for specific conditions.

Doubters of ICPs say that they:

- Take up time which could be spent in other clinical activities.
- Discourage appropriate clinical judgement being applied to individual cases.
- Are difficult to develop where there are multiple pathologies or where clinical management is very variable.
- Stifle innovation and progress.
- Need leadership, energy, and time to be implemented successfully.

Table 2.2 Components of a care pathway for schizophrenia

Standards:

- History.
- Assessment of substance misuse.
- Drug treatment.
- Social functioning.
- Mental state examination.
- Engagement of family and carers.
- Psychological treatments.
- Relapse prevention.
- Risk assessment.
- Patient education on illness and treatment.
- Depression.

routine treatments such as relapse signature training in early intervention teams (Chapter 5) can be tested either from routine data collection or an audit of a sub-sample of notes. One of the advantages of internal audit is that it is experienced by the team as a positive initiative rather than snooping. Testing one's own performance against an agreed target together can be a very motivating experience.

A team audit of clozapine treatment

An AO team served exclusively patients with poorly compliant, frequently relapsing psychotic conditions. About 80% of these patients suffered from schizophrenia, the remainder from severe bipolar disorder. All the patients had histories covering several years. Logically all of the schizophrenia patients would be classed as 'treatment resistant' and the literature suggests that all should have received a therapeutic trial with clozapine. Of these about 30% should respond well and remain on it. We should, therefore, have over 20 patients on clozapine. An audit revealed 2 patients.

We set a target of offering a therapeutic trial to all patients who had not had one in the past. Because of capacity issues we restricted to two starts a month. After one year we repeated the audit. 25 patients had received a trial of clozapine and 12 were now established on it. A repeat of the audit a year later showed that a further 30 had received a trial (we were more confident of the process) and now a total of 25 patients were established on the treatment and clearly benefitting.

Team days and operational policies

Regular team days to review practice and update the team's operational policy are essential. This is also a time to review the audit cycles that have occurred in the preceding year and to take account of new treatments and policy changes (both local and national). The importance of both the operational policy and the process for its local development and agreement is dealt with in specific chapters. It is helpful to consider them as part of clinical governance. The operational policy is mainly to give clarity to the team members about what is expected but also serves vital functions in stating the goals of the team and in giving a framework against which current practice can be judged. Team days give time to reflect on any discrepancy between reality and rhetoric and also an opportunity to think beyond the figures. An audit template can be derived from the operational policy which ensures that team goals can be remembered and regularly monitored. Figure 2.7 is an example of one as used in the IRIS early intervention service in North Birmingham.

Training and supervision

Training and supervision are also vital components of clinical governance. Their importance goes well beyond simply guaranteeing that the appropriate skills are available for the treatments offered. Training and supervision are essential for professional confidence and competence, but also for self esteem and job satisfaction. Without them the heavy demands of work with the severely mentally ill is barely possible. Staff need to be up to date and competent but also to *know* that they are up to date and competent. How much this training and supervision takes place within the team or relies on courses will vary from team to team and is addressed later.

Conclusions

Teamwork has not evolved in mental health by chance. It is the nature of our patients' problems, and the complexities and breadth of the interventions needed to help them

1. **Early Detection and Access**
   - Training programme for GPs and other key agencies in early detection.
   - Written guidance provided to GPs describing how to access services
   - Regular contact in low stigma setting following referral.
   - Alternative strategies adopted before compulsory admission.

2. **Early and Sustained Engagement**
   - Allocation of community based key worker within 24 hours of referral.
   - Home or low stigma settings predominate in contact with client.
   - Sustained and planned engagement for three years before options considered.
   - No clients 'lost to follow-up', unless planned.
   - Failure to engage in treatment does not lead to case closure.

3. **Collaborative Needs Assessment**
   - Multidisciplinary contribution to assessment.
   - Client contribution to assessment.
   - Statement of needs, including symptoms, psychological and social needs.
   - Care plan updated every six months.

4. **Treatment**
   - Use of low-dose or atypical neuroleptics as first time options.
   - 'Streaming' of clients with early psychosis in separate inpatient accommodation.
   - Use of CBT for psychotic symptoms.

5. **Family Approach**
   - Carers involved in assessment process.
   - Provision of psycho-education for family/friends.
   - At least monthly contact with the family.

6. **Relapse Prevention**
   - Early warning signs plan developed and on file.
   - Relapse prevention plan agreed with client.
   - Involvement of family.

7. **Education and Personal Recovery**
   - Psycho-education provided to client.
   - Early vocational assessment and training plan.
   - Availability of vocational recovery infrastructure (links with Further Education Colleges etc).
   - Availability of recovery groups to include recovered clients.

8. **The Basics**
   - Care plan addresses: housing, leisure and income.

9. **Comorbidity**
   - Assessment of substance misuse.
   - Ongoing assessment of depression, hopelessness and suicidal thinking.
   - Assessment of PTSD reaction to psychosis at six months.
   - Use of CBT and recovery groups to promote adaptation to psychosis.

10. **Stigma Campaign**
    - Presence of local strategy.
    - Implementation through primary care, local media, schools and colleges.

(Adapted from IRIS Early Intervention Team. North Birmingham MH Trust)

Fig. 2.7 IRIS Team Audit Summary

that demand it. Mental illnesses are the paradigm multifactorial disorders. They respond to biological, psychological, and broader social pressures and their assessment and management requires understanding and attention to all three spheres. Few of us can master all of these. We have to work together and we have to have differing perspectives if there is to be an added benefit. These professional (and indeed personal) differences give depth to our work but can be a source of disagreement and even discord. Attention to team functioning is a necessity, not a luxury, in CMHTs.

There are common themes that arise whenever team functioning is discussed – team size, generic versus specialist working, leadership, time devoted to meetings etc. They are inevitable because they reflect balances that have to be struck between two ends of a spectrum, each of which can be easily justified in its own right. Generic working leads to smooth functioning, high cohesion and clarity of goals. On the other hand specialist working leads to high skill levels, professional status and therapeutic variety. Both are good but one cannot champion both equally in the same team. The same is true for each of these common themes. While the themes are common to all teams the solutions are not. The differing clinical needs served by individual teams will shift the balance and this is addressed in each of the clinical settings.

Talking about these issues within the team, debating and discussing them, is one of the things that makes the work creative and exciting. There will be genuine differences of opinion and these can be worked through with goodwill. Avoiding conflict at all costs is rarely successful. The trouble taken to acknowledge and sort out differences of opinion and to arrive at a workable operational policy is a good investment. In CMHTs the whole really is greater than the sum of the parts.

CHAPTER 3

Generic adult CMHTs

As outlined in Chapters 1 and 2 the adult CMHT has been the basic model for the development of subsequent, more specialised teams. It was in these CMHTs that role-blurring and skill-sharing first moved out of the rarefied atmosphere of therapeutic communities and captured the thinking of general services. Until recently they were responsible for all the assessment and most of the treatment of adult patients referred for secondary mental health care in the UK. Some form of generic catchment area CMHT was available to well over 80% of the population in 1993 (Johnson and Thornicroft 1993). Their function was the assessment and treatment of any adult patient referred to them, plus support and advice to the GPs who referred to them.

Unlike Community Mental Health Centres in the US (Talbott *et al.* 1987) and unlike the newer specialized teams proposed in the UK NHS Plan (Department of Health 2000), CMHTs had, and have, no explicit template. They were not described and then prescribed, but rather evolved by word of mouth as clinicians tried to find ways of dealing with a changing health care system and rising expectations within fixed resources. As a result there have been many blind alleys along the way and enormous local variation in how they are managed, staffed, and function.

Absence of advocates

With no obvious 'product champion' they have tended to be neglected in much of the debate around service provision. They have also suffered the fate of any uniform public service, namely a vociferous criticism from those who work in them and feel undervalued and exploited (Deahl and Turner 1997). Such moaning and criticism serve a purpose in bonding together those who work in these public services, and are often used to alert the authorities to the need for more resources. Both of these are laudable aims. An unanticipated consequence of such criticism, however, is that CMHTs have acquired a poor reputation among policy makers. Despite the fact that some form of CMHT provides care for the vast majority of patients in the UK secondary services their potential strengths are overlooked because of this emphasis on their problems.

An 'untidy' approach

There is also something 'untidy' about the CMHT, which can make it unattractive to the central planner. This reflects its evolution to fit essentially human, rather than technical, needs. Chapter 2 explores in more detail the ideology and history behind this style of working. This was, in great measure, a reaction against an overly mechanistic and dehumanizing approach to the mentally ill. The CMHT recognizes (indeed celebrates) individual variation both in patients and in staff. It is unashamedly an *interpersonal* undertaking with an emphasis on relationships and personal qualities as well as skills and interventions. CMHTs have been influenced by the 'psychobiology' of Adolf Meyer – although few working in them may know his name (Gelder 1991). He emphasized mental health work more as an open process in which staff and patients were engaged together rather than the identification of diagnoses, which then predicted consistent treatments.

Variation in CMHTs

A consequence of this is that the 'feel' of CMHTs can vary enormously even if their core activities are fairly uniform. The absence of an explicit model, with a firm framework and clearly differentiated tasks and functions, can liberate creativity and encourage empathy but it can also lead to uncertainty, anxiety, and even conflict (Chapter 2). One purpose of this chapter is to provide a draft framework for a generic CMHT from which local, explicit definitions can be developed.

Who is the team for?

The first question one should ask if proposing to set up a new team from scratch is *what* it is meant to do. CMHTs are already set up and are very broad in their remit. *Who they are for* is, therefore, a more realistic starting point.

Age

The separation of adult services from child and adolescent services (CAMHs) (Chapter 7) is established worldwide. Most CMHTs deal with adults '*of working age*'. Thus the lower limit is the age basic secondary education finishes. Over the last 40 years this has risen from 16 years to 18 years in the UK. There is some flexibility (even confusion) about this transition age in different services. Some CAMHs will only deal with 16–18 year olds if they are in full time education, and sometimes local arrangements specify the transition at 17 or even 19 years.

'Hard' or 'soft' transition age?

Some argue against any chronological age cut-off (House of Commons Health Committee 2000), proposing to relate services to the maturity and development of the patient. For individual patients this can make sense. However, for ensuring a rapid, well co-ordinated response, and for planning services, allocating resources, and for advising GPs where to refer, it is quite hopeless. Defining a team needs no doubt about its *responsibilities* – what it must do and what it cannot refuse. An unequivocal age cut-off for responsibility ensures that there is no delay or confusion in providing assessment.

This does not prevent a clinical decision being made, by mutual agreement, for a young adult patient to continue in treatment with a CAMH service or (more often) a mature and very ill 17-year-old to be treated by the CMHT. It is highly likely that this firm age boundary will become less simple with the development of 'young people's' or 'youth' services which are evolving as part of the specialization of first episode psychosis services (Chapter 5).

Need for local clarity about responsibility

The most important issue is to have absolute clarity about the age cut-off locally and for this clarity to be agreed and understood by all stake-holders (GPs, CAMHs, CMHTs, A&E, wards, social services etc). Young people can present for the first time when very ill and there is no excuse for delay and wrangling before their needs are addressed.

Variation in cut-off

The age at which patients transfer to the care of old age psychiatry teams varies inter-nationally, and in many countries there is no specialism of old age psychiatry at all. In the UK the current recommended age is 65 years. This reflects their remit for 'adults of working age'. It underlines the CMHT's commitment to supporting patients' social functioning in employment or education and training. This cut-off, like that for CAMHs, is endorsed by the relevant National Service Frameworks currently being published (Department of Health 1999a). However, not all services do have the same age of transfer and there may be variations, especially around different protocols for functionally ill patients and those with dementia (Chapter 7).

Graduate patients

'Graduate' patients (usually schizophrenia patients who have been cared for by the CMHT for several years) are often controversial. Because old age services are more adapted to patients with dementia, affective disorders, and complications from physi-cal ill-health, they may insist that psychotic patients should not simply transfer auto-matically. Such transfers (unless driven by clinical need) have recently been declared 'ageist' and in conflict with European law.

As with CAMHs services there is no substitute for a crystal clear, mutually agreed and well publicized local agreement. It is not enough to agree on it – it must be clearly recorded in each others' operational policies and widely distributed.

The primary/secondary care divide: severe mental illness

Most individuals with psychological problems in the UK consult their General Practitioner and receive their treatment from the primary care team. Only a very small percentage are referred on to specialist services and an even smaller percentage are admitted to hospital (Goldberg and Huxley 1992). This distribution is often referred to as 'the Goldberg and Huxley filters' (Fig. 3.1). While one might dispute the definition and figures for 'psychological disorder' in the first level few would disagree with the

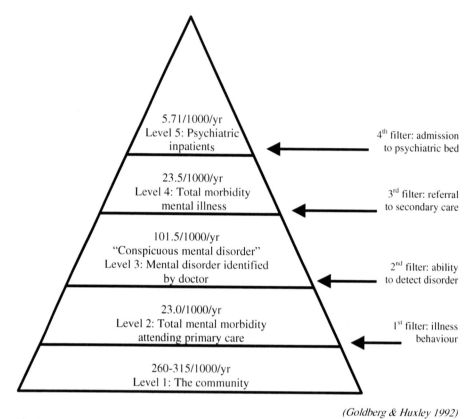

(Goldberg & Huxley 1992)

Fig. 3.1

overall pattern outlined with a narrowing focus as more severely ill patients penetrate further into the system.

'Severe mental illness'

The last 10 years has seen the emergence of the concept of 'severe mental illness' (SMI) or 'severe and enduring mental illness' (SEMI). In the US the term has an administrative status – individuals established by psychiatrists to suffer from a severe and enduring mental illness receive their mental health services free. In the UK the term has no such official status but developed in response to the difficulties in defining mental illness (once a highly controversial concept (Laing 1960; Szasz 1972)) and in response to controversy in the 1980s about whether CMHTs were 'mental illness' services or 'mental health' services.

'Minor psychiatric morbidity' → 'common mental disorders'

To sharpen the distinction 'minor psychiatric morbidity' was originally used to distinguish those disorders commonly treated effectively in primary care. This term was considered to be somewhat dismissive (especially as it was often bundled in with the frankly pejorative term 'worried well') it has recently been replaced by the term 'common mental disorders'. This emphasizes that these are genuine disorders, justifying psychiatric diagnosis, although usually within the competence of non-specialist staff to treat.

The three 'Ds'

Older ideas such as 'psychosis' (often associated with more severe disorders) and 'neurosis' (less severe) had been demoted in psychiatric thinking with their removal from the DSM-III classification of disorders (American Psychiatric Association 1980). Indeed this simple dichotomy never did translate easily into severity – some 'neurotic' disorders were as life threatening and disabling as psychotic ones (e.g. severe depression or obsessive-compulsive disorder or chronic anorexia nervosa). Leona Bachrach (Bachrach 1988) helped clarify the multifaceted concept of SEMI by emphasising chronicity and disability as well as diagnosis with her '3 Ds':

- **Diagnosis** – Psychotic illness, major affective disorder or severe neurosis.
- **Duration** – Minimum of two years.
- **Disability** – Inability to work or fulfil major role function (e.g. parent).

Mental illness and severe mental illness

There is no clear line between 'mental illness' and 'severe mental illness'. The term really indicates a commitment. The early experience of CMHCs in the US and in some CMHTs (especially where direct access was accepted and the distinction between primary and secondary care had been eroded) was that less ill, more articulate patients inevitably absorbed virtually all of the team's resources (Talbott *et al.* 1987). This group actively sought treatment and knew what they wanted. They were also more rewarding to treat as they often recovered quickly. The more ill patients (those with long-standing psychoses such as schizophrenia) were easily overlooked and suffered relative neglect. When a team states that it 'prioritizes the SMI' it is committing itself to ensuring that this neglect is not repeated. It is a statement of intent and not the one that is easily subject to definitions and protocols. Attempts have been made to define the SMI (Slade *et al.* 2000; Strathdee 1998) but they do not seem to have caught on and there is always an escape clause for clinical judgement.

A balanced caseload

While a team may prioritize the SMI for care it must also provide assessment and advice for patients who are not SMI. This is both because the confirmation that an individual has a SMI is itself a specialist function (i.e. the skills and resources of a CMHT are often needed to establish it) and also because CMHTs generally do accept a role in working with moderately ill individuals and those with time limited disorders.

CMHT staff usually overestimate the proportion of their caseload who suffer from psychotic disorders. Although over half the case load of a typical urban CMHT will be of individuals with longer-term psychotic disorders, three quarters of their referrals will be of non-psychotic individuals with milder affective and stress-related disorders (Burns *et al.* 1993*a*; Greenwood *et al.* 2000). GPs must also feel able to refer patients who are not obviously mentally ill so that they can confirm their judgement, and also refine their diagnostic skills. In one representative study (Burns *et al.* 1993*a*) almost 10% of the patients referred to the CMHTs did not reach the threshold for 'caseness' (i.e. were not diagnosed as suffering from any mental illness at all using a structured assessment (Present State Examination (Wing *et al.* 1974)). Even when patients do have moderate or time-limited disorders the GP can profitably use the referral as a second opinion for management. Patients also benefit from the confirmation that their GP is on the right track.

Keeping access wide

Keeping access to assessment broad enough is an essential feature of a well functioning generic CMHT. The lessons of how care deteriorated in large mental hospitals should not be lost on us. Even very good staff can lose sight of the simple human needs of their patients if they are entirely occupied with highly dependent and disabled individuals. Experienced staff often develop very high thresholds for acknowledging distress or disorders. Moving flexibly between patients with temporary mental health problems and intact lives, and those whose lives are totally overshadowed and determined by their illnesses keeps our feet on the ground. It reminds us of the everyday hopes and fears of *all* our patients. Work with a bereaved woman who is struggling with the resultant depression, for instance, can sensitize us to the loss endured by a young man with schizophrenia trapped with the sense of 'what might have been'.

Referral of a 'non-case'

A 28-year-old woman had been weeping in her GPs surgery for the last two visits which were, ostensibly, about her 4-year-old son. The son was fine and the GP worried that the woman was depressed and 'consulting through her child'. He could not figure out what was going on, but knew that the woman's partner drank heavily and there was tension at home. Was he missing a more serious depression? Was there anything the CMHT could do?

The CMHT assessment also started with tears and sobbing but by 10 minutes or so the patient regained her composure. She acknowledged the stresses with her partner (whom she knew was having an affair) but felt she could cope with that "I've never expected much from men – I saw what my dad was like". She confessed herself bewildered about the tears but was clearly tense and guarded. Focusing the interview on her son uncovered that she had recently seen a television programme about Huntingdon's disease and begun to brood about it. She became increasingly convinced that an aunt and her grandmother had been 'odd' and both, she said, had been 'shaky' towards the end of their lives.

She was very annoyed with herself but eventually admitted that she was brooding incessantly on this and had become convinced that she was a carrier and that her son was fated to develop the disorder. Although the psychiatrist did not consider that she suffered from a significant affective disorder he spent time talking through her concerns and agreed to advise the GP. Her GP was informed of these concerns and it was agreed that she would help the patient ascertain the circumstances surrounding the death of her grandmother and aunt. It was a large, local family and the details were easily unearthed and were reassuring. The patient experienced relief from the knowledge and got on with her life again.

Working with less ill patients also helps establish a healthy, realistic appraisal of the prognosis in mental illnesses. It is all too easy to forget, for example, that many patients with schizophrenia make a substantial recovery (Ciompi 1988; Harding *et al.* 1987). Losing sight of this can make us excessively pessimistic and this can easily transmit to our patients undermining their resolve and further demoralizing them. Working with more responsive patients also keeps essential psychological skills up to scratch. We can see gratifyingly rapid results from them, while the same treatments have to be applied over much longer periods and with less dramatic results with SMI patients.

Assessments: routine, urgent, and crisis

Routine (less than four weeks)

A detailed and skilled assessment by a trained professional is one of the most important services a CMHT can offer. Long waiting times for appointments (over 3 weeks) cause sharply rising fail-to-attend rate in outpatient clinics (Burns *et al.* 1993*b*). This study also found that trying to make routine appointments in less than a week was difficult and could alarm patients who interpreted them as implying a more serious condition. Psychiatric disorders are distressing and it is hard to be sure how urgent they are from referral letters. A 4-week limit for routine appointments seems a sensible compromise. To achieve this a team needs to have a degree of flexibility. Referral rates obviously fluctuate, but less than we tend to think. Everyone remembers the one week when the rate doubled, but forgets that, that happened only once in the last 18 months. A useful approach is to check the total referrals for the preceding year, calculate what this means per week and allocate one extra assessment slot in the team's weekly timetable.

Urgent (within the week)

About half the assessments carried out by an inner city CMHT will be considered urgent by the referrer and need to be seen in a matter of days (Burns *et al.* 1993b). Most often these are patients with psychotic illnesses or depressed patients where the GP is concerned about possible suicide risk. If a team has routine new patient slots on 2 or 3 days a week then these urgent patients can often be seen then. They may need assessment at home or the GP surgery.

Crisis (same day)

Where patients are extremely disturbed (possibly needing a mental health act assessment), or where the GP does not know them or is very worried about them, they may need to be seen within 24 hours. This usually means that the patient has become unwell over a longer period and only that day come to the attention of the GP, or that a deteriorating situation has become untenable. Often families will tolerate increasingly difficult and distressing situations until they reach breaking point when the situation then becomes 'a crisis'.

Many teams organize a rota to deal with crisis referrals. We have found this to be a mixed blessing and try and avoid it for three main reasons:

Problems with crisis rotas

1. Wasteful of time (e.g. waiting around if nothing happens).
2. Often staffed by fairly junior members when it is important that very ill people are assessed by experienced staff.
3. Once established it becomes the 'path of least resistance' for non-urgent cases.

CMHT procedures for crisis assessment

Useful standards for crisis assessments are that if referred in the morning they should always be seen the same day by the team. If referred in the afternoon the team will attempt to assess them but otherwise they will be referred to the out-of-hours service (the duty psychiatrist at A&E or crisis resolution/home treatment team) or offered an appointment the next morning if they can wait. Crisis assessments are *only* agreed after direct or telephone contact between the referrer and a senior member of the team. Faxes and messages left with secretaries should not be accepted. The referrer should have seen the patient that day. GPs generally understand this – if it is a real crisis then this is not too much to ask. If the response is prompt and competent then everyone is satisfied.

Assessment procedures:

- Routine: Referral by letter/fax: appointment within 4 weeks.
- Urgent: Referral by letter/fax or telephone: appointment within one week.
- Crisis: Referral by direct contact, patient assessed by referrer that day: assessment same day (by team if possible, duty team if referral late in the day).

Apart from very chaotic inner-city situations the number of crisis assessments generally shrinks rapidly as routine and urgent appointments become more accessible.

Indeed for well-functioning teams out-of-hours crisis assessments (other than Mental Health Act assessments) can become very rare indeed. Although a small part of the work load, these crisis assessments are of enormous importance to carers and referers alike (Johnson *et al.* 2001). Failure to make provision for them will cost a team dear.

Who should do assessments?

Teams vary considerably in their policy about assessments. Originally, assessments were by psychiatrists only – they were 'doctor to doctor' referrals and seen in outpatients departments. With increasing confidence in multidisciplinary working, many teams experimented with assessments by any trained team member. This could be if the GP expressed a preference, for example:

> Her depression is primarily generated by chronic housing problems and I would welcome input from the social worker.

> He has emphatically stated that he won't consider any form of drug treatment for his anxiety state and would like to see a clinical psychologist for counselling.

Allocation meetings

In some teams a decision about the most appropriate member will be made at an 'allocations' meeting. Often this will be determined by the GP's stated preference but not always. It may reflect specific skills within the team or even, simply, preferences by team members for different types of problem. In one team with two equally very experienced CPNs one had a clear preference for short-term 'psychological' interventions and the other for longer-term comprehensive supportive work with psychotic patients. In yet other teams there may be little selection – simply who has the first available slot.

The value of allocation meetings deserves careful appraisal. They can be time consuming, often with detailed discussions about who is most appropriate for a referred patient who (when assessed) turns out to have totally different problems to those indicated in the referral letter. This time could be better used by the team for review of the management of the patient once they have been assessed. If there is to be 'specific allocation' then it is likely to be fairly simple – patients with a psychosis are likely to benefit from some involvement of a CPN, prominent child care issues a social worker, OCD the clinical psychologist and so on.

Effective teams can elect a member to do this sorting without sitting around for an hour a week reading out referral letters and discussing them. A team manager, or any senior clinician, can easily take responsibility for this and the only time required is a few minutes scanning the letters and advising the team secretary who to book them into. Staff often enjoy allocation meetings but a brief trial without them can be revealing when they are not missed and the time used more effectively.

Involvement of psychiatrists

The most controversial issue in CMHT assessments is usually whether they should all involve psychiatrists. There are good arguments for it and good arguments against it. It is worth going through these first before setting out the options. It is essential to try and depersonalize the argument. It touches on very sensitive issues of status and self esteem within teams. It is only too easy to cite a particularly poor member of one discipline and compare them with an outstanding member of another to make a point. There are bound to be teams with relatively weaker doctors and stronger nurses, or vice versa. Indeed there may be overwhelming reasons for adjusting decisions locally. However there are a number of general issues that do need to be honestly faced and thought through first.

The development of the multidisciplinary team has been particularly strong in the UK (Chapter 2), partly in response to the relative shortage of psychiatrists compared to other countries. There is, therefore, a tradition of confident, independent nursing, social work, and psychology disciplines which have taken leading roles in service development and delivery. The arguments around role blurring and an emphasis on a whole-person approach to mental health problems have endorsed a sharing of the responsibility for assessment.

The UK practice of relying heavily on very junior trainee doctors (not the case in countries where training is more university based and routine health care is staffed by trained psychiatrists) has often meant that other team members are significantly more experienced. In Dingleton in Scotland, where role blurring was particularly stressed (Jones 1982), the habit was to pair such novice doctors with more senior non-medical staff for the joint home assessments. Involving non-medical staff in initial assessments is welcomed as a legitimate recognition of their skills and is a part of the job they appreciate. At its most basic it contributes to a happy team.

'Sharing' of staff across the primary/secondary care boundary

Doctors in hard-pressed teams also point out that spreading assessments enhances capacity and certainly some general practitioners have welcomed it. These points warrant careful consideration. GPs have in many instances lobbied strongly for non-medical staff to be 'shared' between the CMHT and the Primary care team. Both formally and informally CPNs (and sometimes psychologists) have been clinically directed by the GP in the same way as practice nurses.

Pros and cons of shared staff

There are good reasons to question the value of this. Although the nurse may welcome the special position as the mental health expert in the GP Practice, they are not funded for that role. Time dedicated to activity in the GP Practice is time and resource lost to the CMHT. It has been argued that '*they are the same patients anyway*' but this is simply

not borne out by experience. The GP's mental health preoccupations are, quite proper-
ly, with the care of large numbers of patients with common mental disorders, not the
SMI. Clinical experience is that such GP-based mental health professionals rapidly
drift from their agreed remit to minor disorders and this has been vividly demonstrated by research in the area (Wooff *et al.* 1988; Wooff and Goldberg 1988). This
Salford study also suggested that there was a demonstrable loss of skill for CPNs disengaged from the CMHT.

Scarce resources

Similarly when psychiatrists encourage spreading the assessments across the team
because of workload it implies either that the team is seriously under-resourced or that
the difficult (and never-ending) task of 'shaping' the local GP referral practice is being
avoided. Working with local GPs to ensure that they understand what a CMHT can,
and can not, do is a crucial part of the job. For most GPs this means encouraging them
to manage most common mental disorders themselves (perhaps with regular support
and discussion with the CMHT) and for a smaller number of GPs to improve their
case detection skills and refer on more patients. Successful teams are generally those
who manage this flow actively in their relationship with the GPs and their practices.
There will never be *'enough resources'* – demand always increases to outstrip supply.

Extent of training

The main argument for psychiatrists being involved in most assessments is the simple
one of that being what they are best trained for. Their training is longer and broader
than other disciplines and, unashamedly, focuses on diagnosis and assessment. If they
are not generally better at assessments then one needs to question why one needs such
an expensive resource. This anticipated competence in assessment is reflected in the
responsibilities and legal obligations vested in doctors. Like other doctors, they are held
responsible for ensuring that patients under their care receive correct treatment.
Legally in the UK all CMHT patients *are* under consultant responsibility although this
is perfectly compatible with a high degree of clinical autonomy (and responsibility) in
who ever is directly treating the patient, irrespective of discipline.

Changing GP preference

GPs have also recently more often expressed a preference for referred patients to be
assessed by trained psychiatrists. This probably reflects our increasingly risk-conscious
and litigation-influenced culture. It may also reflect a recognition that patients in the
public sector should receive broadly similar care to what they get in the private sector.
There (apart from some unidisciplinary interventions for less severe disorders by clinical psychologists) an initial psychiatric assessment is both routine and required.

Trained psychiatrists are very thinly spread in the UK and their levels of contact with
patients are remarkably low by European standards. In response to this one could take

two possible positions. One is that their time should be concentrated on reviewing only complex patients and those with whom other members of the team are having problems. The other is to suggest that investing in the initial assessment is the best guarantee of effective use of scarce resources.

Local decisions

How one decides will depend on the known skills and abilities within the team. If the CMHT is blessed with very highly skilled staff then the argument for only deploying the psychiatrists on complex cases is stronger. Most teams will, inevitably, be average. That means average psychiatrists and average non-psychiatrists. In such a case the advantages of medical assessments for all patients may be greater. Firstly they are more likely to be able confidently to decide in a single assessment that a patient does not need treatment in the team (such assessment approaches are central to medical training, but not to all disciplines). Secondly they are more likely to be able to get the GP to agree with this assessment.

This is a very vexed issue and practice is likely to change only slowly. In local discussions we broadly agreed that every new referral ought to be offered an assessment by a trained psychiatrist. However we set the target at 80% so that clinical judgement can be exercised and so that trainee doctors can continue to get training in assessments. This approach has broadly been endorsed both by the Royal College of Psychiatrists (2000) and by the Department of Health in the CMHT Policy Implementation Guide (Department of Health 2002).

There are also very strong arguments for joint assessments routinely. These can ensure a broad perspective is brought to bear at each assessment and can also provide a continuing stimulus to both disciplines involved to remain alert to alternative understandings. They are more cost effective than they may appear at first sight (Burns *et al.* 1993*b*).

Outreach and home-based care

The CMHT had moved out beyond the traditional outpatient clinic decades ago. CPNs and social workers have always considered the patient's home the logical place for their work. Home-based care has enormous benefits in mental health practice. It ensures that chaotic and disorganized patients (who otherwise often fail to attend appointments) *are* seen. Being visited at home also provides an opportunity to assess the patient in the round. Family members and important neighbours are often met – significant supports that we might not otherwise have asked about, or the patient thought to mention. For very ill patients the state of the flat or house can be an invaluable guide to mental state and general functioning. In UK practice probably around two-thirds of all patient contact by CPNs and social workers is away from formal care settings such as outpatient departments and day hospitals (Burns *et al.* 2000). In a systematic review of all forms of home-based care in mental health, this practice of visiting patients at home was identified as one of the most important characteristics of successful services (Catty *et al.* 2002).

Home-based assessments

First assessments conducted at home have similar benefits. They reduce the risk that the patient will not turn up, ensure that a comprehensive (and perhaps less narrowly technical) understanding of the patients' problems is achieved. Patients also seem to appreciate them and the quality of the interaction is often more equal – they are able to tell you *what they think is important* rather than *what they think 'a doctor or specialist will want to know'*. As an approach it is associated with improved patient satisfaction and overall reduced likelihood of admission (Burns *et al.* 1993*b*; Hoult *et al.* 1984). Time lost on travelling is more than amply rewarded by time saved in missed appointments and resources saved by reduced admissions.

The value of home-based assessments

Heather was 55 years old and had been treated twice in the past for moderate depressive disorders. She had seen a consultant psychiatrist both times in outpatients and had been prescribed antidepressants with follow up shared between the consultant (whom she liked very much) and various SHOs. The first depression had been attributed to marital stress and had been subsequently followed by her husband leaving. The second depression was thought to be due more to her menopause (she said that she had now fully adjusted to the marital break-up) and it took longer to resolve. She was off work for more than 4 months and 'not her real self' for over a year.

The assessment of the third depression, 4 years later, was a home visit by an SpR and CPN. They were given a very similar story of increasing tension and poor sleep followed by hopelessness and exhaustion. Heather was a Roman Catholic, originally from Ireland, and the highly self-critical content of much of her thinking in the previous depressions had been attributed to that. During the assessment her son ('a civil servant in the town hall, still living at home but very settled, no worries' according to the outpatient notes) joined the meeting to express his concerns about his mother. He was emaciated and clearly very ill. Asked about his own health he replied that he had been treated for AIDS for the last 2 years ("Didn't she tell you?"). He attributed his mother's first breakdown to his 'coming out' and the conflict this caused, particularly with his father. The second depression also mirrored a very turbulent period after the break-up of a long term relationship when he was taking enormous risks in his personal and sexual life. He assumed that he contracted HIV during this period.

He insisted that he and his mother had talked through the issues of his gay life-style and that they were both very close and accepting. She emphatically confirmed this – "there is nothing to be ashamed about in such things nowadays". However it became increasingly clear that she blamed herself for the difficulties that the family had in accepting his sexuality and now was devastated by his illness. She insisted that she had never thought to mention it in the outpatient clinic because it was "not important". Both the SpR and CPN felt that she harboured much more guilt about it than she was admitting. Her ongoing treatment (which included antidepressants) included several sessions focusing on her ruminations about her son. He took part in two of these sessions, which were clearly cathartic for both of them and strengthened their closeness. Looking back, when she had recovered, she considered that confronting the tragedy facing her son and her had restored her to her 'real self', while acknowledging that the antidepressants did help with symptom reduction.

Caseload management

One of the most difficult tasks in running a CMHT effectively is to manage the caseload. Without active control caseloads easily grow to the point where the team is overloaded and ineffective. If a team is always full to capacity then effectively it has no capacity. It has no ability to respond in a prompt, coordinated manner to new referrals or crises in its current patients. Constant preoccupation with monitoring an overstretched caseload leaves no time or energy for effective treatments. It has been this difficulty in managing caseloads (especially when an attempt has been made to do so by long waiting lists) that has most often brought CMHTs into disrepute.

For patients with short-term disorders, such as an uncomplicated depression, timing the discharge back to the GP is usually fairly simple. However, there is no simple, easily defined lower threshold for care by a generic CMHT when patients with long-term disorders would be automatically discharged back to their GP. The decision will usually be a clinical one in which the competing needs of current patients are weighed up. To do so effectively requires two preconditions.

Agreed limits

The first of these is a frank recognition of the need for an upper limit and local agreement on what this is. This limit indicates the level where the team can monitor and treat all those it is responsible for, keep up to date with necessary administrative routines and still have 10–15% of its capacity free to deal with the unexpected. This is no small task. It will certainly never be achieved if it is not set as a goal and approached positively. There are two components to such an upper limit.

Individual caseload

There is a maximum number of patients that each member of staff can manage effectively. Obviously this will vary according to the complexity of the patients' needs and the sophistication of the treatments being offered. This has to be negotiated between staff within the team but it is difficult to imagine a situation when the number could be more than 35 patients for a full time professional. This is a number accepted within nursing and now considered too high for more complex or difficult patients. If contact with a patient is less than every 2 to 3 weeks then a team needs to question what they are achieving that could not be provided by well-supported primary care. Whatever the number decided upon it is essential that it is explicit – known to the whole team, talked through and agreed, and written down in the team's operational policy.

Doctors' caseloads

Traditionally doctors have carried variable (and sometimes very high) caseloads of patients they see in outpatient clinics. When we surveyed this locally we found remarkable variation, although the teams were generally equally resourced and had similar catchment areas. There can be little logic to this and so a target maximum of 70 patients was introduced for such patients (many of whom may attend only intermittently for monitoring). At the very least this means GPs can be assured of rough parity of practice across teams.

Team caseload

There is also an overall maximum number of patients who can be efficiently managed by a team, irrespective of how many staff that team has. The whole purpose of teams is to ensure co-ordinated and multi-professional review and input. Long-term and complex patients need regular reviews. Useful contributions to management from different team members requires at least a minimum of familiarity with the patient.

As team size and caseload size rise the balance between transaction times (time spent keeping each other informed about what is going on) and treatment times shifts. A point will eventually be reached when so much time is spent on managing the team activity that nothing useful can be done – or else the team members act effectively as isolated individuals with little useful input from their colleagues.

There is no science to how many patients a single team can manage, but there is an emerging clinical consensus. Local practice has been to insist on an upper limit of 350 (including the doctor's outpatients) and encourage teams to aim for 250. Certainly teams that manage at around 250 seem to be efficient and well appreciated by their local GPs who do not complain of them being excessively restrictive.

Single point of entry

The second requirement for effective caseload management is a single point of entry to the team. Unless there is a common point of entry it is impossible to form an accurate overview of the level of strain or any imbalance in the system. If referrals are coming in and being accepted directly by various team members then it can easily occur that one member is overstretched when another is short of things to do. Similarly the team's capacity to respond effectively to crises and fluctuations in demand can be lost without anyone being fully aware of it and take some action before it is too late. When there are increased referrals and more work, team members can be encouraged to free up capacity by identifying those patients who are now sufficiently well to be discharged back to primary care.

Managing caseloads is not easy. There is enormous subjectivity about which patients are fit for discharge and who is working hardest. Even the best teams will have disagreements. Team management requires recognition of some authority structures (Chapter 2) to resolve these issues even though the preferred goal is always agreement through consensus. The advantage of having agreed explicit numbers is that team members know what is expected of them and manage their own caseload. Only if they fail to do so does it become a team issue.

Systematic reviews

Good quality mental health care is characterised by detailed and comprehensive assessments of patients' problems and needs. Diagnoses are an important, but far from sufficient guide to management. Health, psychological, and social care issues all need attention and their balance will vary between individuals and within individuals over time. Without regular reviews that are, to some extent, prestructured, care easily becomes narrow and mechanical (Wooff *et al.* 1988). The Care Programme Approach (Department of Health 1990) requires a regular review where the patients' needs and the appropriate interventions are recorded clearly along with who is responsible and when they should be reviewed again. Guidance on the procedure changes with predictable regularity but the main message – that patients care should not continue indefinitely without a careful (usually multidisciplinary) review whose conclusions are simply and clearly recorded – remains constant. Few could argue with such a sensible message.

CPA: reality and rhetoric

Because of the long list of recommendations for complex CPA (that the patient and family and GP should be invited, copies of the review sent to almost everybody imaginable, all needs recorded irrespective of whether or not they will be acted on etc.) the approach has often become a battle ground between professionals and policy makers. This is a pity as the idea is common sense and with a little imagination and goodwill can be made to work effectively (Burns and Leibowitz 1997).

Attendance at CPA reviews

The common experience is that GPs rarely attend, and only a minority of patients and families do (although most are pleased to be asked). Patients and families may want to be present throughout the whole review but often more long-term patients ask to skip the presentation of the history and want to discuss the current management. This should not be an excuse to skip over the full presentation. A fairly detailed (structured) review is an essential safeguard against therapeutic complacency or sterility. It simply means interrupting the review to invite the patient to join.

Lengths of reviews

A comprehensive and structured review does not necessarily mean a long review. Long reviews are not only inefficient they are often ineffective – staff benefit by learning to be brief and learning to summarize. About 15–20 minutes is more than sufficient to review even complex patients although this becomes considerably protracted if patient or family are present. If they are to be present then it is important for the key worker to agree and explain the process beforehand. Uncertainty about such simple issues as whether to use first or third person (talking *to* the patient, or talking *about* the patient) in the review can significantly slow things down.

Local guidelines and local paperwork

Most services have agreed local guidelines for which patients should be on enhanced (complex) CPA and what paperwork should be used. It is important that paperwork should support and facilitate clinical practice and not distort it. The CPA, contingency plan and risk assessment forms shown in Fig. 3.2 are samples of the forms used in South West London and St George's Mental Health NHS Trust. We fought long and hard to keep these documents short – a single sheet is always preferred. It forces us to be focused and is likely to be read. Long experience has lso taught us that documents should be completed in the meeting and not left for afterwards. Only then can one be sure that they are up to date and accurate.

ENHANCED CPA/SECTION 117(2) REVIEW (delete as applicable)

Patient's name:	Jenny T	CMHT:
Address:	56 Acacia Avenue	Phone: 0208 XXX XXXX / New patient: YES/~~NO~~ / Date of review: 25.08.03
Phone:	0208 877 XXXX	
Date of birth:	09.09.61	Diagnosis:
GP:	Williams	1 Major Affective Disorder F.32 . 0
Phone:	0208 892 XXXX	2.................................. F __ . __

You must consider the following:

1) Mental health, including indicators of relapse;
2) Physical health;
3) Medication;
4) Daytime activity;
5) Personal care / living skills;
6) Carers, family, children and social network;

7) Forensic history; 8) Alcohol or substance misuse;
9) Cultural factors; 10) Housing/finances/legal issues; **and**
a) make sure **a risk assessment** is done;
b) include: i) **a crisis plan**; ii) **a contingency plan**
i.e. what should be done if part of the careplan can't be
be provided(e.g. the care co-ordinator is on leave or ill)

Assessed needs or problem	Intervention	Resp.of
1. Depressed mood, apathetic and self critical.	• Regular home visits (weekly) to assess mental state and support. • Encourage compliance with antidepressants. • Gentle encouragement to get out - take to shop.	BJ
2. Suicidal thoughts.	• Explore severity (+/- plans) at each visit. • Support mother and husband who are both very scared by suicidal thoughts.	BJ/Cons
3. Daughter's school problems.	• Maintain links with school/class teacher. • Keep family informed of daughter's school functioning.	BJ
4. Plan for recovery.	• When mood brighter encourage support group. • Help her reapply for part time dinner lady post.	BJ

Professionals involved in care:	✓Dr Psychologist CPN OT ✓SW Ward Nurse Support Worker Other
Present at planning meeting:	✓Dr ✓Psychologist ✓CPN OT ✓SW Ward Nurse ✓Support Worker Other

CPA discussed with patient	YES/~~NO~~	Copy given to patient?	YES/~~NO~~	Copy sent to GP?	YES/~~NO~~

Care co-ordinator (print):	Billie Jacks	Phone 0208 877 XXXX
Care co-ordinator (signature):	....	Date of next review: 25.11.03
Job title:	Social Worker	Patient's signature: ....

	Care management? ~~YES~~/NO	Risk history completed? YES/~~NO~~
On Supervised Discharge?	~~YES~~/NO	Relapse + risk plan required? ~~YES~~/NO

Fig. 3.2

CONFIDENTIAL: RELAPSE AND RISK MANAGEMENT PLAN

Name: Alastair W

Categories of Risk Identified:

Aggression and violence	YES/~~NO~~	Severe self-neglect	~~YES~~/NO
Exploitation (self or others)	YES/~~NO~~	Risk to children & young adults	~~YES~~/NO
Suicide and self-harm	~~YES~~/NO	Other (please specify)	

Current factors which suggest there is significant apparent risk:
(For example: alcohol or substance misuse; specific threats; suicidal ideation; violent fantasies; anger; suspiciousness; persecutory beliefs; paranoid feelings or ideas about particular people)

- Ongoing heavy drinking - worse when depressed. Leads to suspiciousness about strangers - particularly other Glaswegians or Irish whom he believes think he is an IRA member and are out to get him. Confronts them often leading to fights.

Clear statement of anticipated risk(s):
(Who is at risk; how immediate is that risk; how severe; how ongoing)

- Risk is to strangers (not staff or family) usually in public houses. Only occurs when mood low and suspicious, often in periods of poor compliance with antipsychotics.

Action Plan:
(Including names of people responsible for each action and steps to be taken if plan breaks down)

- Relapse plan discussed and agreed to increase antipsychotics and report to care co-ordinator when he notices more concerns about IRA - "take more tablets to help you cope with there being lots of them about".
- Attempt to reduce drinking during stressful periods. Usually unsuccessful so encourage him to drink at home, not pubs, at these times and increase visits.
- Advised that if he thinks his life "is at imminent risk" to come to A&E. If presents with this complaint admit to avoid escalation.

Date Completed:	26/01/03	**Review date:**	26/11/03

This risk assessment may contain confidential and/or sensitive information provided by third parties. Such information should not be disclosed to the patient without prior consultation with the informant

---

RISK ASSESSMENT DOCUMENTATION

Client's Name: Georgina A

RISK HISTORY

Give details of any risk behaviour shown by the patient (actual or threatened). **Each entry must be signed and dated**
(E.g. previous violence; weapons used; impulsivity; self-harm; non-compliance; disengagement from services; convictions; potentially seriously harmful acts)

1990-2000:	Over 12 serious episodes of self harm by o/ds and cutting. Twice in intensive care and multiple lacerations.
1997:	Planned extended suicide including her 6 year old daughter (since removed to social services care). Still destabilised by monthly access
2001:	Assaulted SW after access visit. Remains resentful about access conditions.

Fig. 3.2 (continued)

Structured assessments

There are considerable advantages in agreeing a structured assessment as part of any systematic review of long-term patients. Long association can lead to over-familiarity with a patient so that changes in mental state or side effects of drugs are overlooked. Structured assessments also serve the purpose of consolidating the clinical language of the team. When patients are presented along with these results, other members will discuss the ratings and this process helps clarify concepts and calibrate judgements about severity. Commissioners increasingly require structured assessments, both as evidence that patients are getting better and as a quality control measure. With predictable tidiness of mind, efforts have been directed towards developing a single instrument that can be used with all patients. Currently 'HoNOS' (Health of the Nation Outcome Scale) is one such (Wing *et al.* 1999) and is in wide use in the UK and Australia (Trauer *et al.* 1999).

Choice of structured assessment

While HoNOS is admirably comprehensive, covering physical, social, and psychiatric needs there are real doubts about how reliable it is (British Journal of Psychiatry 2000; Amin *et al.* 1999). Not surprisingly, with such wide applicability, it lacks specificity or sensitivity and cannot be expected to alert the professional to minor changes that might otherwise elude them. It may be more useful clinically to use specific scales for specific patient groups. For patients with psychotic disorders the Brief Psychiatric Rating Scale (Overall and Gorham 1962) is short and simple and tracks changes over time with admirable clarity. It is a scale recommended for Assertive Outreach Teams (Chapter 4). For patients with depression the Beck Depression Inventory (Beck *et al.* 1961) is a well-recognised self-report scale that is sensitive to change and often helps stimulate the exploration of problems. For patients who are taking antipsychotics there are a number of scales for measuring side effects (e.g. akithisia (Barnes 1989), Parkinsonism (Simpson and Angus 1970)), and administering these can easily be learnt by all team members, not just doctors and nurses (Chaplin *et al.* 1999).

Note keeping

All professionals need to keep clear, informative notes of their clinical work. In CMHTs there is a long tradition of 'multidisciplinary notes' to reflect multidisciplinary practice. After this clear and simple statement of practice, however, the situation rapidly gets murky. What exactly is meant by 'multidisciplinary notes'? Obviously it means that everyone writes in the notes. But do they all write in the same section, or are there separate compartments for social workers and nurses etc.? In some hospitals there are even different coloured paper for different professions. Are outpatient and CMHT notes the same, and what about community and ward notes? There is such a range of options because there really is no single obvious solution. Current thinking emphasizes the virtues of a single set of notes to cover all eventualities. There are real problems with this as there are with any alternative.

Separate inpatient and community notes

The separation of inpatient and community notes is common because of the need to access previous inpatient notes if patients are admitted out of hours when community notes may be stored in dispersed community mental health centres. The details needed at short notice may also be quite 'state-specific' for inpatient care, such as whether the patient responds badly to a given drug and what interventions have worked well in acute disturbances. Inpatient notes also can become very bulky with long-term patients and too much information can be as unhelpful as too little in a crisis.

Discipline specific notes

The habit of different staff writing in different parts of the notes poses significant risks of misunderstanding. A doctor may look at the last medical entry and be quite unaware of all the changes between that contact and the present which are documented in detail in the occupational therapist's notes or vice versa. For effective multidisciplinary work a consecutive record of contacts is essential. These entries constitute the definitive record, even if more expanded notes are kept elsewhere for other purposes.

Brevity versus detail

For consecutive multidisciplinary notes to work effectively there needs to be some consensus on the style of note keeping – in particular how long entries should be. It is difficult if some team members routinely write nearly a page for each contact and others a couple of lines. A balance has to be struck between the function of the notes as a record of what happened and as a communication of current status and problems to other team members.

Legibility

It goes without saying that detailed notes are of no value if they are illegible. For important documents (such as the CPA record) the advantages of typing are enormous. Where possible it is best to have these forms prepared in electronic format so that they can be typed directly into. This saves time as only that which has to be changed is typed and often considerable parts of the form remain the same. In several countries all notes are typed (often by the clinicians). Perhaps keyboard skills will soon become as necessary as a driving license in community work.

Recording failed contacts

In CMHTs it is essential to record failed contacts. This is partly for legal and administrative reasons but also may raise an alarm. Similarly staff need to record any serious concerns for safety they experience in a visit so that colleagues are warned should they have to do unprepared visits in a crisis or to cover sickness.

Inpatient care

Not all CMHTs take responsibility for inpatient care. Indeed, internationally this form of continuity of care is rare. In the sectorized system which evolved in the UK (and simultaneously, though less comprehensively, in France (Kovess *et al.* 1995), Chapter 8) this continuity of care has generally been the case. The advantages in terms of pragmatism and the avoidance of excessively theoretical practice have been outlined above. In simple, day to day, practice it is associated with much better bed management – i.e. patients are discharged more promptly, length of stays are generally shorter and early readmission rates are lower.

Continuity of care and safety

Continuity across this boundary also has an important bearing on safety. The Confidential Inquiry into suicides and homicides identified the first week after hospital discharge as the highest risk period for suicide (Department of Health 1999*b*). The rate of suicide in this immediate post discharge period was significantly raised in NHS patients admitted to private sector beds. This raised risk reflects the lack of familiarity with relevant issues (both patient and context) during the transfer between two teams at this most vulnerable period.

Benefits of transferring care

There can, of course, be advantages to having two perspectives on a problem. Being able to 'hand over' a patient, even if only temporarily, is sometimes necessary where relationships are strained and both sides feel exhausted and pessimistic. GPs talk openly about the use of secondary services on occasions to give them respite from long-term, stuck relationships. The Italian mental health care system seems to tolerate lots of team changes for patients to everybody's apparent satisfaction. There may be some merit in this arrangement but it is better for teams to acknowledge it for what it is rather than avoid it by having an expensive and inefficient duplication of teams.

Well-functioning teams are able to recognize and discuss when an individual therapeutic relationship has become stuck or dysfunctional and arrange an internal transfer. At the team level some form of pairing to allow for second opinions, or even permanent or temporary swaps of patients, can work well. This requires trust, and if one-half of the relationship begins to exploit it, it will falter.

Primary care liaison (and primary care liaison teams)

CMHTs can only really succeed if they establish an effective relationship with the primary care teams who refer patients to them and accept them back from them. Even when patients are under the care of CMHTs they remain actively involved with their GPs. The SMI have a consultation rate with their GPs which is higher than average (about 8 visits a year (Kendrick *et al.* 1994)) and GPs are the health professionals most frequently in contact with long-term mentally ill individuals. They are also the ones (along with CPNs) that patients would choose to contact. Most of this contact is for repeat prescriptions, certificates, and minor physical problems rather than focused mental health care. Nonetheless most GPs have an important place in the care of patients and that care is invariably 'shared care' although of a relatively informal kind.

Psychiatrists have been involved for several decades in helping GPs deal with complex psychological and psychiatric problems in their patients. Initially this took the form of 'Balint' groups where a psychiatrist (usually with a psychotherapy interest) explored with a small group of GPs the unconscious and relational issues involved in management of individual patients. The interest was as much in the GP understanding their own responses to difficult patients and the psychiatrist rarely ever met the patient (Balint 1968).

Shifted outpatients and shared care

Balint groups have become less common and were replaced by mental health professionals spending sessions in primary care settings where they could do assessments without patients having to go to secondary care settings. This form of overlap, often referred to as 'shifted outpatients' grew out of good interpersonal relationships between GPs and CMHTs and by the early 1980s a quarter of English CMHTs and a third of Scottish CMHTs were regularly spending some time in primary care premises (Strathdee and Williams 1984).

A South London GP, Ben Essex, pioneered a formalized shared care with his local CMHT (Essex et al. 1990) and Ian Faloon's Buckinghamshire project provided 'secondary' mental health care in the GP setting using only primary care notes (Wilkinson et al. 1995). Shared care is an attractive concept in mental health but generally the evidence does not favour it (Warner et al. 2000). Clarity of responsibility is of paramount importance as 'splitting' can so easily occur. Simple confusion about 'who agreed to do what' can arise causing poor outcomes for the patients and bad feelings all round.

Liaison meetings

Probably the most common form of primary care liaison currently consists of regular, scheduled meetings between members of the CMHT and Primary Care Team (Burns and Bale 1997). How many attend from each side, how often they occur and their format all vary. Large group practices (which can be individually responsible for half a local CMHT's referrals) may find it valuable to have monthly meetings with all partners present and the whole of the CMHT. Smaller practices with fewer common patients may prefer a 'link worker' where one CMHT member of staff comes regularly to the surgery. Often this is the CPN who may combine liaison with some direct patient contacts.

GPs are less enamored of long, structured meetings than mental health staff seem to be. Most successful meetings are only 30–40 minutes, usually with only a very rudimentary agenda. A list of the practice's patients currently in care with the CMHT is a useful prop and can be quickly run through together and problems discussed.

Discussion does not have to be restricted to patients currently in shared care but usually relates to those the CMHT have had some direct contact with. Potential new referrals can also be discussed.

Discussing problem patients serves other purposes than simply refining management. It is a much more effective method of defining what the CMHT can and cannot do than any number of protocols. Honestly discussing therapeutic limitations together dispels myths and clarifies processes. It also can build trust and goodwill – especially when both teams have to accept that some patients have both of them beat. Simply sharing the frustration and problems of dealing with impossible patients removes the 'them and us' feelings that can otherwise so easily develop.

Primary care liaison teams

The development of more specialized teams for delivering secondary mental health care affects the roles and remit of the traditional CMHT. Where crisis and home treatment teams, assertive outreach teams and highly developed rehabilitation community support teams exist the CMHT will have less of a focus on the SMI. One possibility is to emphasize the development of skills in primary care liaison and, in particular, the provision of enhanced psychological treatments within primary care. This approach is still experimental but clearly has important implications for the range of skills and activities deployed in CMHTs. An optimal, or durable format for such teams will have to await longer experience.

Conclusions

CMHTs have evolved to meet a broad clinical need with very limited resources. They have suffered by not having a clear description of their functioning and roles. This latter is not surprising – the boundaries between those who do and do not need their specialist input are neither prescribed nor easily described. Clinical judgement and consensus remain at the centre of their effective working and inevitably involve a high degree of subjectivity.

CMHTs evolved into their present form simultaneously with developments in therapeutic communities and share many similarities in practice and ideology. Both emphasize a sharing of skills, and a degree of role-blurring which balances generic with specialist working. Both stress the importance of staff as whole people, relating honestly to patients well beyond the narrow confines of diagnosis and treatment. They aim to harness the full creativity and potential of all staff members. Patients understand their disorders in terms of their own personal narrative and CMHT staff need to encompass this.

Children of the 1960s

CMHTs and therapeutic communities are both 'children of the 1960s' and as such are ambivalent about authority. Inevitably there is tension and some conflict. Most often this is creative but occasionally can become locked and then needs confronting.

Lacking an identified model and product champion they have often received a poor press – much worse than their performance deserves. They do, however, need clarity of purpose and active management if their potential is to be fully realized and for them to survive in an increasingly accountable health care system. The achievements and efficiency of a well-functioning CMHT are, however, an example of a highly evolved, fit for purpose, system that commands genuine admiration.

CHAPTER 4

Assertive outreach teams

Origins of assertive outreach

Assertive outreach teams are the most established of the specialist teams in UK, US, and Australia. Their history starts with the development of case management in the US in response to deinstitutionalization (Intagliata 1982) and took off with the landmark study of PACT by Stein and Test in Madison, Wisconsin (Stein and Test 1980). This study compared the outcome of allocating half of patients destined for admission with relapse of their severe mental illness to an experimental team of case managers and letting the other half follow the standard care that was offered at that time. The PACT team (Programme for Assertive Community Treatment) was composed of nurses, mental health aids, and social workers with input from psychiatrists. They took on only 10 patients each and were committed to doing 'whatever was necessary' to encourage their patient to stay well. In practice this meant that they ensured that the patients took their medicines, and gave them intensive help with social functioning and generally sorting out their lives.

PACT

PACT is a form of clinical case management. Initially case managers had an administrative function ('brokerage case management'), linking discharged patients with the care they needed but not providing it themselves. However, this soon changed to 'clinical case management'. Clinical case managers are trained healthcare professionals who combine the administrative and co-ordinating roles of brokerage case managers with direct clinical care. Solomon classified clinical case management into three main groups with PACT as one example of 'full support' (Solomon 1992).

Types of case management

- ◆ Brokerage case management:
  - • Expanded brokerage
- ◆ Clinical case management:
  - • Personal strengths model
  - • Rehabilitation
  - • Full support (including PACT)

Initially Stein and Test called their approach 'Training in Community Living' (TCL) as they expected a period of such input to equip their patients to survive in society with chronic psychotic disorders – a form of social skills training. Unfortunately the funding for their innovative service ran out and (luckily for our understanding of effective outreach) they had to stand by and watch as all the gains in the 14 months of the study were lost. They realised that their approach was not so much a *training* as a community *support* programme, hence the change in name.

Success of PACT

Demonstrated superiority

PACT became enormously influential internationally. There are probably two reasons for this. Firstly, the Stein and Test study achieved remarkable reductions in hospitalization but also improvements in clinical and social functioning and also patient and family satisfaction (Stein and Test 1980). It was also judged to be cost effective – i.e. to cost no more than standard care despite clinical superiority. It depends on how the calculations are made (Weisbrod *et al.* 1980) as to whether the Madison service cost the same as standard care or slightly less. However, John Hoult's replication in Sydney (Hoult *et al.* 1983) was unequivocal in its finding of improved outcome for less cost. Not many new approaches start with such a ringing endorsement.

Clarity of definition

The second reason for the impact of the PACT approach is probably the clarity with which it is described. Both the treatment principles and the service specification are explicit and fairly concrete. The five components of their model are set out below and four of these still actively inform current ACT teams. Freeing the patient from pathological dependency was a concern in psychiatry at that time, both as a response to the experience of institutionalization observed in mental hospitals and also deriving from theories current then about dysfunctional family relationships causing or exacerbating schizophrenia (Bateson *et al.* 1956; Fromm-Reichmann 1948). This is a tenet of PACT which has faded but can be replaced with a commitment to support and encourage maximum personal independence for the patient. The original concern with pathological dependency has contributed to some of the earlier doctrinaire disputes over the 'whole team' approach (Burns and Firn 2002*b*). The model articulated now is strikingly simple, robust, and comprehensive. Not high-tech, but very patient-focused.

PACT programme principles

- Provision of material resources for patients.
- Fostering patient coping skills.
- Supporting patient motivation to persevere.

PACT Programme Principles *(continued)*

- Freeing patient from pathological dependency relationships.
- Support and education for those involved with the patient.

Specification of the service went beyond simply describing the model and philosophy which is the usual level of detail in services reported in studies. Stein and Test were much more specific and described the individual aspects of practice that they considered essential to their approach.

PACT core components

- Assertive follow-up.
- Small caseloads (1:10).
- Increased frequency of contact (weekly to daily).
- *In vivo practice* (treatment delivered at home and in the neighbourhood).
- Emphasis on medication.
- Emphasis on engagement.
- Support for family and carers.
- Provision of services within the team where possible.
- Liaison with other services when necessary.
- Crisis stabilization and availability 24 hours a day, 7 days a week.

Very few mental health treatment approaches are so well-described or so well-known. The approach has been widely replicated and studied (Marshall and Lockwood 1998; Solomon 1992). There are over 75 scientific studies of PACT or PACT like services in the literature (Mueser *et al.* 1998) and they constitute the majority of home-based studies that have been conducted in mental health (Catty *et al.* 2002).

Model fidelity

The precision of ACT description has even given rise to scales to measure 'ACTness', (e.g. Teague *et al.* 1998) and in the US organizations such as CARF (The Rehabilitation Accreditation Commission) undertake assessments and accreditation of a range of mental health services including ACT. The spread of ACT in the USA and Canada has utilized a modified 'franchise' approach ensuring a similarity of approach. In the UK the National Forum of Assertive Outreach services is less strict but does aim to encourage greater consistency of practice across its members. While this clarity of definition has been a major advance in mental health services innovation it has occasionally given rise to sterile and unhelpful arguments about whether a team is a 'real' ACT team. Such arguments generally presuppose much more certainty about the effective components of the approach than is warranted.

Who is assertive outreach for?

Psychotic patients

PACT is the model *'evidence-based service structure'*. However it is important to recognize that this proven effectiveness is with a fairly clearly defined patient group. It has also been defined in a specific service context of which more will be said below. PACT has been shown to reduce the need for hospital care and produce equal or sometimes better outcomes only with patients suffering from psychotic illnesses (Marshall and Lockwood 1998; Mueser *et al.* 1998; Solomon 1992). The approach does seem to have merit even when these psychotic patients have other problems such as homelessness or drug and alcohol abuse (Drake *et al.* 1998) although the only published trial with offender patients failed to demonstrate an advantage (Solomon and Draine 1995a). Assertive outreach approaches are being tried out with different patient groups (e.g. those with personality disorders, those with learning difficulties and challenging behaviour), but currently there is no evidence for this and such innovative teams need a period of observation and then evaluation before the practice is widened.

Hard to engage patients

Discussions about who assertive outreach is for often obscure the more important issue of being clear which *treatments* are to be provided by the proposed team. Assertive outreach is often referred to as if it were an effective treatment in itself. It is not – it is simply a service structure to deliver treatments to a specified group of patients. If there are no effective treatments delivered then there will be no benefit.

This crucial understanding of assertive outreach is particularly obscured when it is being proposed for 'hard to engage' patients. Although, when planning a team, we often pose the question *'who is AO for?'* in reality we should be asking *'what is AO for?'* What treatments will we be able to deliver with this set up that we cannot deliver without it? Len Stein has frequently said that there is no point in having small caseloads unless the contact frequency is raised; and no point in frequent contact unless those contacts contain assessments and monitoring; and no point in those assessments if they are not associated with providing effective treatments and rehabilitation. In other words there is no inherent virtue in, for instance, 'engagement' – the purpose of engagement is to provide the opportunity to negotiate and provide effective treatments whether they be pharmacological or psychosocial.

The therapeutic relationship

Nevertheless assertive outreach is very appropriate for hard to engage patients. Engagement does not mean simply making contact with patients. It refers both to this and to the long-term maintenance of the relationship – working on engagement is *always* part of the job. A strong therapeutic relationship is a powerful determinant of how well a patient will do, whether with drug treatment or any form of community care (Priebe and Gruyters 1993). Assertive outreach, because of its wide remit, allows the key worker to cement and build the relationship by attention to those things that matter most to the patient. Obtaining benefits, securing accommodation, accompanying to leisure pursuits all make clear to the patient that we have their best interests, not just their symptoms, at heart. Such shared activity and patient-centred planning helps with mutual understanding and through that engagement and cooperation in treatment.

The therapeutic relationship has always been highly valued and considered in psychotherapy. Assertive outreach teams are often somewhat sceptical about psychodynamic psychotherapy but a revaluation of the importance of such thinking is under way in routine mental health practice (McGuire *et al.* 2001). The patients referred to assertive outreach teams (see below) make great demands on staff and some understanding of the stresses in the therapeutic relationship, and how to manage it, are essential.

'Revolving door' patients

Most of the research evidence targets patients with well-established and severe psychoses who suffer frequent relapses. In some ways this is circular – if reduced rehospitalization is the main outcome measure then the approach cannot be tested on patients who are not regularly using hospital. In effect this means mainly younger schizophrenia patients in the first 15 years of their illness when their mental state is still very fragile and fluctuating, and severe bipolar patients. In practice it also means patients who are generally poorly compliant with their treatment – failing to take maintenance medication regularly is a major cause of relapse. Clinical experience bears out these research findings. Assertive outreach has its most obvious benefits in patients who suffer regular relapses with florid positive symptoms and not surprisingly improved compliance with medication is one of the most important contributions the team can make.

Negative symptoms

The Wandsworth service initially took on a small number of stable but very disabled patients. These were predominantly isolated, self-neglecting schizophrenia patients with marked negative symptoms and fixed, low grade delusions. The quality of their lives was so poor that we invested extensively in trying to sort out their accommodation, self care, social contacts etc. The results were very disappointing. Indeed most of these individuals found the increased level of contact distressing. Any improvement in their material circumstances was more than outweighed by the experience of 'intrusion'. Once again the experience confirms the need to have some effective treatment to offer to justify the intensity of contact.

High risk and 'difficult' patients

The intensity of contact in Assertive outreach means that patients can be closely monitored and signs of relapse noted early. As a consequence treatment changes can be initiated promptly either to prevent a relapse or, if need be, to arrange admission. This is particularly important in a small group of patients whose relapses (though perhaps not very frequent) are particularly severe and pose significant risks either for the patient or others. Severe bipolar patients, particularly, fall into this category as their relapses can be abrupt and dramatic and they may destroy vital relationships or lose jobs as a result. Short compulsory admissions for such individuals should not always be seen as a failure. Similarly patients who behave in a self-destructive or dangerous manner when ill need extra protection as the consequences of even a few days' illness can be disastrous.

Assertive outreach teams should prioritize such patients. Not only does the close contact protect by prompt action, but it also enables a better, more personalized risk assessment. Close familiarity with the patient can make the case manager more sensitive to earlier warning signs. Regular contact is also protective of the staff-member because they are not going 'blind' into a visit to someone they have not seen for two or three weeks who may already be floridly unwell.

'Difficult' patients

Overlapping with the high-risk group is a group of patients who, for want of a better term, can be called 'difficult'. Often these are patients with a fearsome reputation within the hospital and service because of their behaviour when ill. They are often threatening, assaultative, or simply unpleasant to staff (condescending, insulting etc.). As a result they often disengage soon after discharge to the mutual relief of both parties. Contacts with the service will have been fraught and often aversive (compulsory admissions with police involvement, intensive care wards, and often medication administered against their wishes). Many feel angry and hurt by these experiences, while others (particularly some bipolar patients) feel embarrassed by the memory of how they behaved, hence the rapid disengagement. Such patients do very well indeed with assertive outreach. Regular contact, not driven by clinical crises, enables staff to get to know the patient more as a real person and vice versa.

Having a restricted caseload legitimizes the case manager to spend time with the patient when they are at their best and can begin to discuss and understand the processes which lead up to frequent relapses and can then plan strategies to avoid or reduce them. For most of these patients it is the first opportunity for health care staff to get to know them and like them. Genuine affection and respect are much more effective in engaging and supporting such patients in the community than attempts at control. This process is not, however, rapid. With our bipolar patients it took about two years to note the difference. The first signs are often in how case managers discuss the patient. Initially it is usually in terms of anxiety and risk, but this gradually goes over to positive advocacy with ambitions for improvements in their life-circumstances. Obviously it cannot always be possible but most mental health staff are generous and tolerant individuals and can find something to like in almost anyone. Detailed reviews can help by reminding us of how awful life has often been for these patients and by actively encouraging a positive take on the current situation.

Compulsory admissions

High risk and difficult patients generally have a history of compulsion in their care. Over two-thirds of the Wandsworth ACT patients have histories of multiple compulsory admissions and most of current admissions are on section. There is no real contradiction in striving for a collaborative and respectful therapeutic relationship and the use of the Mental Health Act when needed (Burns and Firn 2002c). Most assertive outreach services will be expected to take on patients whose care is characterized by higher than average frequency of compulsion. Being able to work through the feelings generated by compulsory admissions and still maintain a trusting relationship is one of the necessary skills of assertive outreach workers.

Team structure and routines

Team members and size

Assertive outreach teams need to be multidisciplinary to provide comprehensive care. They need nurses, psychiatrists, and social work input as an absolute minimum. There is good evidence that full integration (not just part-time peripheral attachment) of a psychiatrist within the team is a requirement for success (Catty *et al.* 2002). US teams stress the value of vocational counsellors and substance abuse specialists but these disciplines are not well-developed in Europe. Often members of the team with a special interest shoulder these roles (e.g. Occupational Therapists are often well equipped for vocational work and nurses are increasingly trained in appropriate family therapy skills).

The size of the team is important. In urban settings teams are larger and serve up to 100 patients (generally considered the maximum that can be coped with efficiently) whereas in less morbid settings teams may serve as few as 50 patients. The Mental Health Policy Implementation Guide recommends caseloads of up to 90 for urban teams and up to 60 for rural teams. Teams with less than five case managers have real problems managing because of vulnerability to sickness, covering holidays etc., and also because the reduced flexibility can make safety and responsiveness difficult (see below). To function well a team needs to meet face to face regularly and all members need some familiarity with all the patients discussed (Liberman *et al.* 2001). This puts the ceiling on team size at about 12 full-time staff (Child 1977). Part-time staff are clearly often a major resource for AO teams but given the need for close communication (especially around unstable, potentially dangerous patients) there are special problems associated with having too many.

Case managers

The backbone of the assertive outreach team is the case manager. The case manager has a restricted caseload. Originally this was recommended at a maximum of 1 : 10 but this is rarely adhered to and up to 1 : 15 is common. The case manager has an extended key worker role, which involves co-ordination of care and liaison and advocacy, but also has a central core of direct care delivered to his or her patient. This role involves both general mental health interventions (e.g. monitoring mental state, supervising and administering medicines, assessing side effects) and more specialized interventions dependent on skills (e.g. family therapy, CBT for delusions, motivational interviewing). It also involves a broad sweep of psychosocial and rehabilitative interventions (e.g. skills training, group work) plus essential social supports (e.g. obtaining benefits and accommodation, ensuring adequate physical health care and nutrition). AO case managers would expect to see all of their patients at least once a week, and probably twice a week for most. Some patients will need daily contacts for brief periods for specific interventions (see below) but contact once or twice a week is essential if the care provided is not to be entirely medical or crisis-driven.

Internationally AO case managers are usually nurses (common in the UK, Italy, Scandinavia, and Australia), or social workers (common in Germany and some US teams). In the US and some Australian teams graduates in social or health related courses but without further professional training are common. Given the severity of disorders in AO patients most teams are reluctant to have non-professionally trained case-managers taking key worker responsibility. The Care Programme Approach in England (Department of Health 1990) requires a professionally trained key worker although a non-professional can work with the patient under the supervision of the key worker who holds that responsibility. Non-professional key workers are becoming increasingly common in the UK with the establishment of AO teams in the voluntary sector. How this will work out in practice is still to be seen.

Stratified skill mix

There is currently debate about whether the case manager should take responsibility for fairly simple, but time consuming, tasks such as accompanying the patient to the social security office or tidying up the flat. Some have proposed that less skilled mental health workers should undertake these tasks thereby leaving the case manager to get on with the more technical parts of the job. The pressure for this mainly reflects concerns about the cost of AO staff and also the shortage of such trained professionals. Undoubtedly this stratified approach can work well but may demonstrate a misunderstanding of the model and history of AO.

It is precisely in the broad range of activities that the therapeutic relationship is established and there is an opportunity for patients to redefine their stance towards services. Cutting out the 'low-tech' parts of the job deprives AO of much of its unique potential to turn around dysfunctional engagement with services. Certainly there can be a sharing of such routine tasks. In the Wandsworth ACT team the user worker (who is not professionally trained and cannot carry CPA responsibility) shoulders a large part of the routine medicine supervisions and visits to social services etc. However this is *shared not segregated*. The proposal to stratify tasks very rigidly tends to come from non AO-staff who see the more generic approach as a threat to their professionalism. It is rare to hear it advanced by experienced AO case managers.

User workers

Individuals who have themselves suffered from mental health problems have been very successfully employed in assertive outreach teams. Indeed Solomon has reported from the US on a service where all the case managers in the team were service users (Solomon and Draine 1995*b*). The close working relationships of these teams should ensure adequate and close supervision and support.

The user/worker (or consumer worker – there are several possible terms) is particularly well placed to encourage patients to persevere with medications, being able to draw on their own experience and therefore having high credibility. They also have little problem in identifying with their patients and acting as more effective role models than other staff whose achievements may seem altogether too remote. They also are a concrete embodiment of the philosophy of AO teams – that patients are whole individuals with strengths and weaknesses, not just diagnoses. Having a service user as a colleague in the Wandsworth ACT team has been an enormously successful experience. In England such staff cannot take full CPA responsibility and have to work alongside professionally trained staff.

Gender and ethnic representation

As in any mental health team it is important to ensure that staff reflect the ethnic spread of the patient group they serve. There is no strong evidence for ethnic matching of individual patients and case managers, but the team needs both to understand the world view of their patients and to be perceived by their patients as understanding it. This would be difficult if there was a very stark ethnic divide. Similarly there is a need for both male and female case managers. It is a common mistake to believe that dangerous or threatening patients can only be managed by male staff. Quite the opposite is the case as female staff generally elicit less confrontation. However there are times when men are needed, and times when women are needed. Few teams can survive without at least one female nurse as many female patients (particularly from ethnic minorities) will not accept close personal care such as depot injections from males.

Medical staff

PACT quality standards are quite specific about the need for trained medical staff as part of the assertive outreach team (Allness and Knoedler 1998) and a systematic review of home treatment services for mental health problems (Catty *et al.* 2002) identified the presence of psychiatrists as integral members of the team as crucial to success.

A full-time psychiatrist for a team with 100 patients is proposed in the US and this seems about right. Obviously the psychiatrist is necessary for many of the interventions that are currently restricted to medics (e.g. prescribing, organizing involuntary treatment when needed) but their role should be much more than that.

There is little sense in having a psychiatrist as a case manager although some have tried this. Doctors are rarely able to offer the level of consistency and input required in this model. However they can contribute substantially to comprehensive assessments and ensure that the treatment side of the 'treatment/rehabilitation' balance is not forgotten.

Status

Psychiatrists have an important role to play in relationships with the outside world where their status can still (perhaps regrettably) achieve action when case managers' inputs have failed.

Avoiding 'drift'

It is certainly very easy in a successful assertive outreach team for the focus to drift exclusively to the social and psychological aspects of care, and doctors have a crucial role in being alert to this. Paradoxically they are more likely to achieve this if they are fully signed up to the psychosocial goals of the team and can demonstrate skills in this area (Liberman *et al.* 2001). This identification of the psychiatrist with the whole model is picked up in Catty's systematic review where it was not the *availability* of medical time that made a difference but their *integration* in the team.

Social workers

The emphasis on integrated health and social care in this model makes it difficult to run such a team without a trained social worker as a member. The rapid and extensive skill sharing that characterizes the approach soon results in most of the case managers becoming proficient in many traditional social worker tasks (e.g. housing applications, benefits). However many patients have very complex social care needs (such as appointee-ship to manage their finances) and social workers have greater access and status within social services hierarchies and can advocate more effectively for patients there than other team members.

There also remain specific powers restricted to social workers (e.g. Mental Health Applications, some child protection issues, some expensive residential provisions) and familiarity with the system is also invaluable in less specific areas (e.g. knowledge about local resources and funds). Because of the very time consuming nature of these tasks social workers usually have a reduced caseload. This is important as inflexibility in responding to pressing tasks could lead to complications, extra work, and bad feeling. In the Wandsworth team the social worker has a two-thirds caseload (8 instead of 12 patients). The balance between generic and specialized work has to be thought through with the social worker as with any other team member, and it is important that the whole team 'owns' this balance.

Occupational therapists

As in generic CMHTs occupational therapists make excellent case managers. Some seek jobs in Assertive Outreach teams because they want to extend their professional activity beyond that which is traditional within OT. Others find the fit for their OT skills in this team approach particularly gratifying. Certainly the more structured and reflective thinking that they bring to the use of self and the organization of time and leisure for patients is an enormous asset. The existence of a well-developed theory, with practice that spans widely differing patient groups, is a significant advantage (Kielhofner *et al.* 1998). OTs are often members of assertive outreach teams in the UK whereas in the US Vocational Rehabilitation counsellors are more common. Not surprisingly, given their training and skills, OTs often take on a responsibility for vocational services within UK teams. With their groupwork training they also often take a significant lead in family support groups and leisure groups. Vocational rehabilitation, family support, and leisure are, however, core aspects of assertive outreach functioning. Careful thought has to be given to how much the OT works as a generalist and how much as a specialist – probably more so than with any other team member.

Clinical psychologists

The potential contributions of clinical psychologists to assertive outreach teams will be only too obvious – CBT for delusions and hallucinations and with depression, behavioural analysis and rehabilitation programmes for stuck or challenging patients etc. Unfortunately, in North America, Australia and Europe Clinical Psychologists have tended not to work in such teams. The reasons are probably more to do with professional culture than with financing (although this is often advanced). The issue of balancing generic with specialist working (which is a sensitive one for all mental health professionals) appears to dominate the debate. This, along with the long-standing rivalry that exists between psychiatrists and psychologists, means that for all practical purposes clinical psychologists are not involved in assertive outreach. Hopefully this will change.

Hours of operation

Assertive outreach teams invariably work some form of extended hours – they are not 9am–5pm, office hours, teams. In the literature 24 hour services, 7 days a week are recommended, indeed proposed as the hallmark of such teams (Hoult 1986; Stein and Test 1980). There is, however, little evidence that successful AO teams really do work 24 hours a day 7 days a week. Most use local duty systems for night times or offer a very restricted back up service – often simply a telephone advice system. This makes good sense.

Close supervision means that sudden crises are unusual. What can be offered in the dead of night is very limited and the resource implications of a 24-hour service soon make themselves obvious to teams. Giving time off in lieu of night duty leads to fragmented provision and the alternative of paying staff overtime rates based on the assumption that they are going to be awake and working is both prohibitively expensive and misleading. Very little happens for such teams in the night. A local audit in Wandsworth found only four calls in 3 months of 24-hour availability. Three of these were from a patient for whom an effective contingency plan was available for the Emergency room and one was a patient we had been trying for some time to admit and which was achieved smoothly by the duty psychiatrist and social worker. The inconvenience of regular on call from home soon becomes irksome to trained and experienced staff if nothing happens. Even worse if they are called for trivia.

Weekend working

Extended hours have, however, proved their worth and few teams work only 5 days a week. Seven day working is particularly useful for patients who need supervision of medicines. Similarly for those who seem rather shaky, and where a team would otherwise have admitted them over the weekend to be on the safe side, can benefit considerably from brief monitoring visits at the weekend.

Weekend working may be a reduced service. The Wandsworth team has only one staff member available at weekends. Despite this there was a significant reduction in short admissions in unstable patients after moving to 7-day working. Because there is only one member of staff on the visits are almost entirely planned ones – the proportion of 'crisis' visits is even lower than during the week. Staff conduct an average of about seven visits a day at weekends as opposed to 4–5 a day during the week.

The emphasis on planned visits at weekends is a policy decision driven essentially by safety considerations although unscheduled visits are conducted if the case manager knows the patient and the situation. Usually these are arranged at a 'safe' location such as the ward or the Emergency room. The weekend can also be an excellent time to catch up on paperwork if things are not busy. Only over zealous orthodoxy can justify running a completely full service at weekends. Liasing with other agencies is rarely possible as they are closed and patients also want their week to have a rhythm with more leisure during these two days.

Shift working

Most ACT teams work two shifts thereby providing a service from 8am to 8pm with an overlap in the afternoon. The advantages of extended hours are obvious. It means that one can work with families who have jobs, it facilitates leisure activities such as taking patients to the cinema or evening classes and it can mean that daily supervised medicines can be planned for later in the day (particularly useful with clozapine which makes patients drowsy).

While this is the dominant model in Australia and very common in the US we have not found it so useful in the UK. Firstly there are issues of safety in large cities. Many AO patients live in areas of the city where it is simply not safe to visit after dark. Obviously this is regrettable for what it signifies about patients' quality of life, but it is a fact. Also only a third (at most) of our patients have families to work with, so that focus is limited. Shift systems complicate forward planning of treatment programmes, which can be confusing to patients.

Wandsworth ACT found it more effective to work office hours with a stated requirement in the job description for case managers to work up to one evening a week flexibly depending on clinical need. We require the case manager to take time off in lieu and not to collect more than one month's time back (i.e. about two days). In truth, for most, it works out at less than this.

Joint visiting at short notice when patients are thought to be relapsing and there may be a risk is an essential capacity in AO teams. Being able to arrange this without it either being a hassle or resented is the hallmark of a successful team. A critical mass of sufficient case managers can be reliably maintained when all work 9am–5pm but may be more difficult in a shift system when the whole team is only present in the afternoons.

For large teams with an unstable and shifting patient group the shift system may be best. However it is important to analyze the real needs of your patient group and neither deny necessary services nor provide availability when it is unnecessary and unused. This is very much an area to avoid dogma and to audit practice.

Team meetings

Like other multidisciplinary mental health teams AO teams need to have a regular system for reviewing assessments of new patients, periodic and systematic reviews of current patients, staff supervision and management structures, and some form of away-day to review policy and team strategy (see Chapter 2). Handover meetings and structured reviews have a defining place in the smooth running of AO teams.

Handover meetings

This is a daily meeting lasting about 20–30 minutes. Its purpose is to keep all members of the team fully up to date with current issues. The format is simple with the team leader simply going through the whole list of the patients and reading out their names. If there is nothing to report nothing is said, but if there are issues of concern or recent developments these are briefly mentioned. Usually this is by the key worker but not necessarily so. For instance when patient A's name is mentioned one week the key worker may respond:

> Yes, I haven't been able to make contact with him for over a week. His mother's worried about him and I think he may be relapsing. Could everyone keep an eye out for him?

Another time when the same patient's name is mentioned a different case manager contributes:

> I've seen him coming and going from Dean's flat. Dean says he's had a row with his mum about drinking but is fine. Dean said he would try and get him to be there for my next visit and I'll let you know.

Often new and enthusiastic case managers slow down handovers – either because they are anxious about their caseload or because they interpret contribution to the meeting as a sign of activity. Some sensitivity is needed in helping new team members get the sense of the threshold for contributing so that the meetings do not become unwieldy.

Tasks are allocated if any staff are off sick (e.g. a patient was due to be accompanied to the well woman clinic by her key worker who is off with flu so another case manager has to be identified to step in). Problems can also be raised at this meeting – particularly issues of safety and risk where one case manager may need someone to accompany them on a visit to a patient who has become threatening.

Using 'whiteboards'

Handover meetings are used to co-ordinate the tasks within the team. In large, busy teams it is essential to have fail safe prompts to make sure that vital visits are not over-looked. The need for simple, reliable systems reflects the 'team approach' with shared responsibility for the care of individual patients. It is even more marked in Crisis Resolution and Home Treatment teams (Chapter 6).

Whiteboards have become indispensable for this purpose. Regularly recurring tasks which are shared in the team, or intensive management of patients in crisis (especially daily visits for supervised medication), are written up on these boards. It is much easier to forget a planned intervention if it is with 'somebody else's' patient. Even if the key worker takes responsibility for all of them, high frequency contacts should be indicated so that the team is alerted to cover in the event of sudden absences.

Whiteboards clearly can only be used in offices that offer a degree of confidentiality. Even when there is no patient access to them it is important not to use surnames because of casual access (e.g. cleaners, maintenance staff, etc.). They easily get messy so energy spent organizing a permanent grid is worth it. Equally it is important to clean and rewrite it often – washable marker pens take some cleaning off. Block capitals are also worth striving for.

Figure 4.1 represents the whiteboard used in the Wandsworth ACT team. Where the key worker is responsible for all the daily visits an arrow through the days is used for simplicity. Names of key workers indicate the days they are visiting. For weekends no names are used as the member of staff on duty does all the visits. It would be too messy to write in the purpose of the visit – this is in the notes and is discussed in handover. A significant number of patients receiving regular visits do so because of directly supervised clozapine. These patients are indicated with a 'c' against their name.

Where patients pose a significant risk and need joint visiting (Jerry B and Hayley M in this example) both names are added. As only one person is on at the weekend joint visits cannot be provided, so the Sunday contact received for Hayley M is scheduled for A&E after a telephone call.

Patient		Mon	Tues	Wed	Thur	Fri	Sat	Sun
Carmel C	c	Judy ———————————————————→				Pete	V	
Patrick G		Andrew	Pete	Andrew	Pete			
Rory R	c	Pete	Pete	Bob	Pete	Pete		
Marsha K		Bill ————————————————————————→						V
Ann Marie L	c	Helen	Becky	Becky	Helen	Becky	T	T
Jerry B		Caroline & Bill		Caroline & Bill		Caroline & James		
Patricia M	c	Anne ———————————————————→						
Nikki D		Andrew	Andrew		Andrew		T	
Edward B		Vic			Vic			V
Hayley M		Vic & Andrew	Vic & Andrew		Vic & James			T
Peter W	c	James ———————————————————→					V	V
Mandy H		James		James				
Keith M	c	Helen ——————————————————————→					V	V
Jennifer K	c	Pete ———————————————————————→						
Robbie D	c	Andrew ——————————————————————→					V	T

c = Clozapine   V = Visit   T = Telephone call

Fig. 4.1 Supervised Medications/Daily Visits Board

Clozapine boards

AO teams who target severe psychotic illness will inevitably accumulate a high proportion of treatment resistant cases. These will require clozapine treatment and a major
advantage of AO in their care is that treatment adherence can be significantly improved
by supervised administration as described above. Missing blood tests are a real
headache with such patients as they can often result in temporary interruption of the
treatment and the need to titrate the dosage again.

A white board is enormously helpful in tracking when clozapine bloods are due
(Fig. 4.2). In this the Wandsworth ACT team use numbered weeks rather than the dates
and indicate with a star when the bloods are due. In the example given, when week 40
(the current week) is completed the heading is altered to week 44, and after the next
week 41 becomes 45. It is very simple once one does it. Some patients attend the clozapine clinic (C) but many have their bloods taken at home (H) by their key workers
(O'Brien and Firn 2002), but these are always done on the same day of the week to
avoid uncertainty or problems with pharmacy. Like the daily visits board, the clozapine
board prompts the team if anyone is away sick or on holiday and has not arranged
cover.

Patient	Bloods	Frequency	Key worker	Week 43	Week 40	Week 41	Week 42
Karen P	C	4	Peter	*			
David A	H	4	Andrew			*	
Hazel F	C	4	Becky			*	
Hannah L	C	4	Becky		*		
Aaron E	H	4	Becky				*
Kevin D	H	2	Anne		*		*
Jerry B	C	4	Anne	*			
Ann Marie L	C	4	James	*			
Glenn M	C	2	James	*		*	
Elsie L	H	4	James		*		
Roy S	C	2	Judy	*		*	
Jake P	H	2	Judy		*		*
Eric M	H	4	Peter			*	
Daisy D	C	2	Peter		*		*
Basil J	H	2	Bill	*		*	
Sandra M	H	1	Bill	*	*	*	*
Monica L	H	2	Andrew	*		*	
Hazel O	H	2	Andrew	*		*	
Iris L	C	1	Anne	*	*	*	*
Joseph M	H	1	Judy	*	*	*	*
Robert P	H	1	Bill	*	*	*	*
Matthew K	H	1	Helen	*	*	*	*
Edward B	H	1	Helen	*	*	*	*
Rebecca W	H	1	Caroline	*	*	*	*
James F	H	1	Caroline	*	*	*	*

H = Home   C = Clinic

Fig. 4.2 Clozapine Monitoring Whiteboard

Timing

In teams that operate shift systems the handover is particularly important – indeed its rather inaccurate name reflects its origins in the handover between nursing shifts. In these teams it usually takes place at lunchtime or early afternoon – at the start of the late shift. In teams with no shift system it is usually conducted at the start of the day. In the Wandsworth ACT team we moved it back from 9.00am to 9.30am because several patients have to be visited very early (i.e. before 9.00am) if we are to be sure of catching them in. Rather than having the meeting routinely disturbed by such late arrivals the new time of 9.30am was set. This gives team members some time before the meeting for informal discussions about patients and writing up notes. It is not an excuse for continued lateness and the handover meeting really does highlight the importance of punctuality in an AO team. A 20-minute meeting that starts 10 minutes late is simply not acceptable. Effective team working generally needs punctuality but nowhere more so than at these brief fixed points.

Clinical review

CPA reviews

AO patients have complex needs and require a formalized review of their progress and treatment at fixed intervals. It is important that they are not only reviewed in depth when there is a crisis of some sort. Similarly it is essential that the review is comprehensive and structured so that assumptions are revisited and myths dispelled. In the UK there is a requirement for such regular reviews for CPA (Department of Health and Social Services Inspectorate 1991). In some teams these reviews are incorporated into the multidisciplinary review meeting (this is the practice at the Wandsworth ACT team) whereas in others CPA reviews are conducted separately with only those staff involved with the patient included. The advantage of this is that the review can be longer, which is often very appreciated by the patient and carers who attend. The disadvantage is that it is not informed (indeed challenged) by the combined wisdom of the whole team.

Whether or not the periodic review also serves as the CPA review it is optimal to try and involve the patient and family in the review along with other important stakeholders such as the general practitioner. It is rare for general practitioners to attend but patients and their families may often want to come and should be encouraged. As discussed in Chapter 3 the managing of these reviews requires some flexibility and tact.

The need for structure

The value of structured assessments of clinical and social functioning as part of the review is even more important in AO patients than in most CMHT patients. This is because the close working over long periods can lead to overfamiliarity, with an attention to details that leads to a failure to recognize aspects of the basic illness. For instance it is very easy for a team to become preoccupied with sorting out the increasingly complex social chaos of a patient without stopping to realize that they are all consequences of his or her hypomania that has been coming on gradually. A routine requirement for assessing mental state as part of the review process is invaluable. The Wandsworth team used the BPRS (Overall and Gorham 1962) and a composite scale to assess medication side-effects (Chaplin *et al.* 1999). Both these can be easily administered by the case manager although letting the junior doctor conduct the assessment now and then can act as a useful check on reliability.

Crises and problems

As well as regular structured reviews this meeting also serves as a chance to discuss problems and crises as they arise. Experienced team managers learn to prolong some of these discussions so that more than one alternative solution can be considered and through that encourage more creative thinking. These discussions can sometimes be much more effective and vivid training experiences for the team than academic case conferences. Promoting a culture of openness, where more junior staff feel able to express anxieties and concerns, and receive support and helpful suggestions rather than be made to feel failures, is one of the team leader's central tasks. It is essential both for learning and for safety.

Documentation

AO teams will inevitably collect a core set of paperwork that they use for all patients. The most common are set out below.

Routine documentation

- Care Programme
- Risk assessment
- Contingency plan
- Relapse plan

AO patients will all need to have a formal care plan which is up to date and comprehensive (see Chapter 3).

Risk assessment

A formalized risk assessment is also necessary – even if this records that risk has been considered and is not judged to be significant. Risk assessment is currently a controversial issue, with unrealistic expectations of what can be achieved reflected in detailed check lists of no proven worth. Staff express concerns that if they record risks they will be held accountable for any subsequent disasters ("You wrote that you were aware of the risk. Why didn't you admit the patient until the risk was passed?"). On the other hand if risks are not identified and recorded then will we be considered negligent if a disaster occurs? Damned if you do, damned if you don't. However, it would be foolish and unprofessional not to consider and document the risk history for AO patients. Where there are known triggers and risk factors (e.g. alcohol, preoccupation with some well-circumscribed delusions) these need to be carefully documented. The Wandsworth ACT team resisted an exhaustive check list approach and favoured a more narrative style with enough detail to set the risk in context.

Contingency plans

Contingency plans are essential for AO patients as these are likely to be 'revolving door' patients who, despite close follow up, will turn up in Accident and Emergency rooms or police stations. A sample form (as used in the Wandsworth ACT team) is shown in Chapter 3. There are four essential features of managing contingency plans:

Success with contingency plans

- Keep them simple
- Target carefully
- More than paper
- Review regularly

Keeping it simple

It can be tempting to fill contingency plans with details of history and management and relapse signatures. This is a mistake. Contingency plans need to be simple and constructed with a view to the situation where they are used. They will most often be used by a duty doctor facing a significantly ill patient, often with the presumption of admission being an urgent necessity. The clinician's judgement will determine the outcome, the contingency plan is not intended to replace that judgement but to inform it. Only those facts which are essential to a decision but not likely to be volunteered by the patient should be included in the contingency plan:

Has presented repeatedly at A&E threatening suicide. Has never acted on threats. Usually this is when he has run out of money and has no food at home. Ask about current situation and reassure that he will be visited early the next morning. Offer 100 mg chlorpromazine for sleep. Try and avoid admission.

Advice *(not instructions)* should be given clearly with the reasons for that action equally clearly and succinctly expressed. A telephone number on which to leave a message is vital. Duty doctors are reluctant to make disposal decisions that rely on them making contact with services several hours later – they like to feel they have wrapped up the problem before moving on to the next one. Remember that it is the clinician's responsibility and the wording of contingency plans should be sensitive to this. Clumsy or dogmatic contingency plans will backfire and are bad for professional relations.

Targeting carefully

All contingency plans will usually be distributed to agreed services: the local A&E department (including adjoining hospitals in some urban settings), the home treatment/crisis resolution teams, the General Practitioner and duty nurse for the inpatient services. However individual patients may have their own patterns of help-seeking behaviour and this should always be considered when preparing and distributing the forms. Some patients have strong attachments to particular wards where they have been admitted before and simply will turn up there irrespective of how comprehensive your local provision is. A Wandsworth ACT patient routinely crossed London to seek admission at the hospital where he had been treated 20 years previously for his first breakdown. They received regularly updated contingency plans. Simply writing that patients should be transferred directly to an agreed place for assessment is easily said but far from easy to do.

Police and social services

A small number of patients may regularly end up at the police station. Most mental health professionals are uncomfortable about leaving patient details with police but for a selected few it may be essential and saves endless problems. Where this is done the wording of the contingency plan will need to be carefully thought about and individually composed – the person reading and using it is likely to have very limited understanding of mental health:

> Jason suffers from a long-standing mental illness. He regularly comes to police attention by wandering into offices and libraries etc. and haranguing staff incomprehensibly. He appears quite threatening and frightening but means no harm. *He has never assaulted anyone.* These episodes are not malicious and soon calm down. His key worker (telephone no …) will come and collect him from the station and stay with him till he is settled.

Some patients regularly go to social services offices (particularly those with unresolved feelings about childcare issues) or to social security offices or housing departments. There are important ethical issues about how free one should be with distributing information and each must be decided on a case-by-case and need to know basis. The factors to consider include the consequences of the wrong decision being made in the absence of information, the likelihood of the patient turning up and the reliability and responsibility of the agency being informed.

More than just paper

Nobody is going to take a piece of paper seriously in a difficult situation unless they know who it is from and whether that person's opinions can be relied upon. There needs to be some level of personal contact with where contingency plans are sent. For routine recipients (wards, A&E, duty doctors etc.) a regular system of face-to-face contact ensures that those receiving the plans understand the team (what it can offer, how it works, and what sort of people it comprises). For duty systems this contact needs to be at least every six months because the junior staff who usually run them keep changing. Such routine meetings not only inform the duty staff, but they also confirm in the most concrete manner the commitment of the team to what is in the contingency plan. "This is a team that really will turn up." Where the plan is going to a more one-off setting (e.g. the housing department, police) then it is essential that it is delivered, not sent. This gives an opportunity to explain the rationale behind it and the working methods of the team. Without such an input you can be sure that the plan will be ignored.

Regular reviews

Contingency plans (just the same as risk assessments) need to be updated regularly. Making a routine to update all such paperwork along with the routine CPA review is the best policy. Often nothing will have to be changed but the date and date for review. It makes sense for the updated form to replace the old one (even if the wording is the same) in the patient's notes to confirm that it has been updated. It is not necessarily good practice to send such unchanged forms routinely to all other agencies. We have found that they get annoyed with unnecessary mail and most prefer only to be informed if something is changed. It should be made clear in the face-to-face meetings (and perhaps in the introductory documentation) that the plan is regularly reviewed at least every six months. Without such an assurance such plans are of little value.

Inpatients

Hospital admissions are an essential component of the care offered by AO teams. They are not a failure. Studies of ACT teams show that they do not significantly reduce the *number* of admissions although they can and should reduce the *length* of admissions (Marshall and Lockwood 1998; Mueser *et al.* 1998). There are a number of ways in which admissions are handled. In the US, some parts of Australia, and much of the UK, the patient comes under the care of another team when admitted. In many countries this separation between services for community and inpatient is the norm. In the UK it is not routine but may be necessary in AO teams because the small number of admissions makes comprehensive care impractical or inefficient. In such a case admissions may either be through the crisis resolution and home treatment team as in the North Birmingham approach (Minghella *et al.* 1998) or to the relevant CMHT (Kent and Burns 1996).

Although handing over inpatient responsibility may be time efficient for small Assertive Outreach teams it carries with it all the disadvantages for patients, and scope for conflict, inherent in such divided responsibility (Chapter 2). For larger teams, who are likely to have at least 4 or 5 inpatients at any one time, the advantages of continuity of care and consistency of message by managing its own beds may outweigh the time saving of not having to conduct ward rounds etc.

Inreach

Even if the inpatient care is provided by another service the assertive outreach team needs to keep close contact with its patients and remain actively involved in management, particularly discharge planning (Burns and Guest 1999). It is through this that assertive outreach reduces inpatient stays. Assertive outreach case managers are not superhuman and may, like any other mental health professional, breath a sigh of relief when a patient has been admitted after a particularly stormy patch. The tendency is to give themselves a well-earned rest with that patient. However that is not what AO is about and maintaining the relationship is essential. Wandsworth ACT sets an 'inreach' contact target of 3 times a week – one more than our community target of 2 times a week to counteract this understandable human response. It is justified on the grounds that inpatient visits are shorter and much less comprehensive – though this is not always so. It also is a very important message to the inpatient staff who easily feel 'dumped upon'.

Respite admission units

All that has been said about admissions holds equally if the patient is admitted to a routine acute admission ward, an intensive care ward or (as is increasingly the case) a crisis house or respite admission unit. These small units generally take less disturbed patients (few can manage patients on section) and are more domestic in character. They are dealt with in greater detail in Chapter 5 (Early Intervention Teams) as they play a particularly central role in the care of first onset patients.

Referrals and discharge

Stein and Test advocated a 'no-discharge' policy for assertive outreach teams (Stein and Santos 1998) and this is often quoted as optimal policy. This is very questionable. Assertive outreach is recommended for individual patients on the grounds of their exceptional clinical and social needs – not simply on their diagnosis. It is in the nature of severe mental illnesses that they settle down in most individuals – this has been repeatedly and convincingly demonstrated for schizophrenia (Ciompi 1988; Harding *et al.* 1987) and observed, but not so thoroughly documented, in bipolar affective disorders. Only a very small proportion of ACT patients are over 55 years old. This reflects the natural history of psychotic disorders with both a clinical settling from severe fluctuations to a more stable disability, and also a reduction in the social chaos driven by the disorder. In comprehensive mental health services where less intensive care can be provided (e.g. by a good CMHT) it makes sense to transfer them when the clinical and social needs become less pressing – just as CMHTs transfer back to primary care when patients have settled or recovered.

Referrals

Assertive outreach teams need to have a clear target patient group and this will inform the referral process. This is dealt with in detail at the start of this chapter and needs to be clear within the team and made clear to those in a position to refer. It is argued in some settings that all patients who meet the agreed criteria should be taken on by the team without individual assessments. There are strengths to this argument. Firstly it is fair – the AO team cannot be accused of favouring one CMHT over another. Secondly it protects the AO team from an accusation of avoiding the very difficult patients (the hostile, dual diagnosis patients who are rarely easy to work with) and of 'cherry picking'. This is an accusation that has been levelled against some research teams (Coid 1994). Lastly it honestly reflects our lack of certainty (beyond the basic characteristics outlined above) about which patients are going to do well with us.

Assessment

It is still important to assess each referral individually. This allows identification of immediate needs and often the choice of keyworker. Where the patient is an inpatient it means that the team can make a plan to become involved in discharge planning and handover. This initial assessment also allows for some prioritization. Sometimes the needs of a more recently referred patient may require immediate engagement (i.e. someone about to be discharged from the ward or whose long-term CMHT key worker has just left). Some degree of queue jumping is inevitable. Being too rigid about the order of acceptance of patients is unhelpful. However, these judgements need to be made carefully and sensitively if bad feeling is not to result. In the Wandsworth ACT team the assessment is made jointly by the team leader and the keyworker thought most likely (from the written referral letter) to take on the patient. Doctors are not involved in this assessment.

Waiting lists

With fixed caseloads there is a likelihood that new referrals may have to wait to be taken on by the team. There are problems with waiting lists in mental health. It is a common experience that once a patient is agreed for transfer to another service then the 'holding' service becomes just that – *a holding service* – with little active commitment to improvement. Patients should not be kept waiting more than about three months. If there is a flood of referrals it may be better to identify the 2 or 3 with a likelihood of being accepted soon and turn down the others. The gateway criteria for an assertive outreach team outlined above are likely in urban settings to be too inclusive for the capacity. Clinical judgement must be exercised. It is essential that such judgement is both consistent and transparent.

Inpatient referrals

Patients accepted for assertive outreach are generally given a minimum period of attempted engagement irrespective of how it goes. The Wandsworth team guarantees to persevere for 12 months come what may. However there are special issues with inpatient referrals. Sometimes patients will be discharged to the AO team when quite unfit for discharge, even sometimes with parts of the history not being disclosed. Where a local rehabilitation team has a long waiting list the CMHT may refer the patient inappropriately to the AO team who rapidly realize that the patient is incapable of independent living irrespective of the level of support and care. One strategy is to stipulate clearly that should patients accepted by the AO team from inpatient care who need readmission within 2 months then this *may* be back to the referring team not the AO team and acceptance of the referral reconsidered. This does not *have* to be the case, and often the AO team will deal with an early readmission and carry on. It is a defence against 'dumping' which unfortunately sometimes does go on.

Discharge from AO

Well defined admission criteria are the norm in AO teams but few think through discharge criteria. Unless there are effective discharge criteria teams will soon silt up and not be able to accept new patients. Effective working of AO teams needs a proactive approach to caseload management. If they do not, unacceptable situations will arise where more seriously ill patients are cared for in the CMHTs than in the AO teams whose clientele may have settled after some years of intensive input. Case managers are often understandably reluctant to consider discharge for patients who are now doing very well but only after years of struggle. Sometimes the patient themselves will ask for discharge when they feel better, but this is rare.

10–15% turnover per year

The Wandsworth ACT team, now that it is fully established, experiences about 10–15% turnover per year. This means the discharge of one or two patients per month with new patients to take the place. The team has evolved a system of triggering a 'discharge' review if the patient has not been admitted for 2 years nor has experienced a significant episode of deterioration during that time. Definitions of such a deterioration are not precise. Clinical deterioration is generally fairly simple – it is a relapse with intensification of positive symptoms accompanied by a need for significant treatment changes (often manipulation of the drug dose or contact frequency). It is considered that such a clinical relapse would have led to an admission were the patient not receiving assertive outreach. Sometimes the relapse can be more social than clinical (e.g. a period of increased drug use or of disengagement and behavioural change) but this is just as important in assessing readiness for discharge.

Although this absence of relapse triggers a discharge review it need not end in discharge. Other factors may override. Some patients are so dangerous when they relapse that the risk cannot be taken until some more significant and 'permanent' qualitative change has occurred in how they function. For others one may judge that the engagement is so-intense that disturbing it runs a very high risk of disaster. Sometimes, when it has taken 5 or 6 turbulent years to get there, 2 clear years simply does not seem enough. Clinical judgement must be allowed in this setting – there is no highly developed technology available and no place for dogmatism.

Failure to engage effectively

AO teams are meant to 'add value' to a patient's care. There is a growing body of clinical knowledge about those who do and do not benefit. Handing back to a CMHT when the patient has not benefited can be difficult. Teams say 'If you can't help what do you expect us to do?'. The unpalatable answer is that no service can be sure of helping everyone. Despite best efforts, some patients simply fail to engage and can only be cared for during their relapses. It then can be a tricky clinical question whether or not to continue investment in following up and attempting to monitor the patient. Is this really a worthwhile use of resources if it has no discernible impact on the nature or frequency of relapses or the individual's quality of life between relapses?

Successful improvement is an indication to discharge back to the CMHT as out-lined above. There are other reasons to consider discharge, which reflect a matrix of engagement and treatment:

Levels of engagement: consideration of discharge

- Absolutely no contact.
- Contact achieved but no treatment.
- Treatment achieved but no engagement.
- Successful treatment but no change in attitude.
- Successful treatment and increased autonomy.

Failure of contact

Some patients effectively elude contact no matter how hard we try. They simply do not want to see us and take active steps to avoid us. They may refuse to answer the door when we arrive. They may shout at us to go away or pretend to be out although we may know that they are there. Some make a point of being out or even leaving home and finding new lodgings.

Failed contact

Jason is one of a large West Indian family with several members afflicted with psychosis. His aunt and his elder brother both committed suicide. He is a talented artist and has sold some of his paintings. His diagnosis has varied over the years but most recently has been that of schizoaffective disorder. Relapses are long and severe, with florid hallucinations and elaborate delusions about pollutants being absorbed through his skin. He is usually admitted agitated and overactive and, with treatment, settles becoming profoundly depressed when he blames himself for his brother's suicide. In this depressed phase he has made 2 serious suicide attempts. When recovered, however, he always absolutely refuses any contact whatsoever – politely but unshiftably.

After 15 months and 2 compulsory admissions the ACT team had to acknowledge that they had failed to make any contact with him between inpatient spells. The relationship fostered as an inpatient did not carry over to the community setting. Neither did persistant visiting bring any success. There was a hope that the ACT service would facilitate earlier (possibly voluntary) admission but this did not happen either. After negotation the CMHT reluctantly accepted him back.

These present difficult ethical balances. Just how persistent should we be? The Wandsworth ACT always follows up for one year making a minimum of about one attempt a week. It is, of course, different if a patient meets with us and clearly and explicitly demands to be left alone. In such cases an individual's 'right to be ill' eventually has to be respected. There is little gained in occupying a scarce ACT slot with a patient who is never seen. They should be discharged back to the CMHT. Indeed many

CMHTs argue that keeping such patients 'on the books' is unhelpful and that they should go back to the GP if they refuse any intervention.

Contact without impact

For some AO teams 'engagement' is the goal. Staying in contact for prolonged periods may be all that is feasible and all that is attempted. The expectation is that this relationship will eventually mature and treatment (perhaps from a more clinically orientated team) will then be accepted. This undoubtedly does happen. The time scale will vary considerably depending on target populations (e.g. it would be longer for groups such as the homeless) and the team ethos.

Most AO teams consider contact and engagement to be steps to treatment:

> You aim for *contact*, in order to *monitor*, in order to provide effective treatments and rehabilitation.
>
> (Len Stein, Personal Communication)

How long does one persist with engagement which does not lead to treatment? The following case history describes a patient where engagement and contact have been maintained for several years with neither demonstrated benefit or acceptance of treatment. While hospital treatment is successful, contact has neither made it possible to intervene earlier nor to achieve this without compulsion. It is probably, overall, a better use of resources for failure to be acknowledged and transfer back to the CMHT organized. A frank recognition is needed that there has been no added benefit to the patient and that the CMHT's task is no easier.

Engagement without treatment

John had suffered from schizophrenia for nearly 30 years. He came from the West of Ireland and was generally a shy reclusive individual, a devout Catholic, although not a church goer. On referral to the AO team he had been admitted at least annually for the last 10 years. Admissions were always traumatic and involuntary. Usually the police found him dishevelled and wandering lost in London. He became fearful and aroused when approached and force was always necessary. He responds well to antipsychotics in hospital and settles. He refuses treatment out of hospital. While he recognizes his illness is schizophrenia he insists that God gave it to him for a purpose and will cure him when the time is right.

The AO team have now had regular contact over 4 years. He is polite, accepts visits but refuses treatment or 'interference with his life'. He absents himself and goes wandering when he relapses. His admissions have not changed in frequency or character. Should he remain on the AO case list?

Treatment without engagement

Paradoxically it is possible to achieve effective, if limited, treatment without developing engagement. As the following case history shows, patients may eventually, grudgingly accept the inevitability of maintenance medication but refuse any more meaningful contact. In most cases this frosty relationship thaws over time and more comprehensive treatment is established. Sometimes it does not. Although the AO team's persistence may have been essential in establishing it there may be no need for them to continue. Certainly if this is simply a depot, or filling up a dosette box weekly, then handing back to the CMHT is probably sensible.

Effective treatment without engagement

Alison is now a widow in her late fifties. Her husband managed the medicine for her schizophrenia, until he died 6 years ago. After his death she stopped taking any treatment and refused contact. Admissions (always difficult) became twice a year rather than every 2–3 years. They also involved the police having to break in when her sons reported her deterioration – often messy and traumatic events.

The AO Team established her on oral antipsychotics by daily supervision. Getting this established required a couple of further admissions. Visits were brief and surly with her taking the tablet and refusing to talk to us. After nearly 2 years of this she agreed to transfer to a depot and is now visited only weekly. Not a particularly 'rewarding' therapeutic experience. However, she has now had nearly 3 years out of hospital and her sons are delighted that she (and they) can get on with their lives again.

Treatment success with and without change

Effective treatments can be established which result in real and tangible improvements in our patients' lives. In the best scenario patients, benefiting from both the treatments and the rewards of a stabilized social situation, start to take responsibility for their own illness management. These are the unequivocal successes and soon transfer back to the CMHT when they are relapse free.

Relapse on transfer

Some patients, however, despite these improvements, do not want to take more responsibility for their illness. It is perfectly possible for some patients to respond extraordinarily well to AO care but remain dependent on it. Sometimes this can be a rude shock when all seems well, they are transferred back to the CMHT and promptly relapse. It is often unclear whether what they miss is the structures and procedures of AO care or whether those procedures have permitted a quite different kind of therapeutic relationship with their key worker. The loss of that relationship may be a real blow if it is not possible to replicate it in the CMHT.

Balancing support with challenge

Pragmatism is the order of the day in both these situations. AO teams may continue for extended periods despite their input appearing mechanical and limited. If the risks of relapse are great, or there is no sign of the patient's dependency reducing, this may be the only safe solution. This can often be very unrewarding for the keyworker and needs to be sustained across the team. Currently only by challenging the dependency in some patients is their capacity for greater autonomy revealed and the risk of transfer has to be contemplated.

Our judgements can (and will) be wrong in some instances. Some patients we think have completely outgrown us relapse on transfer, and others who we think will find the transfer difficult flourish. It is always a careful clinical decision for individual patients. Without confronting these decisions the team will ossify and become ineffective.

Handover

Having decided that a patient is ready for discharge after several years in an AO team the process of discharge has to be worked through. The patient has to be prepared for the change, the receiving CMHT (or other service) needs to be prepared and even the case manager needs time to work through the disengagement. Wandsworth ACT use 6 months as the usual time scale for handover. At the very minimum the AO team must have scaled down the level of input to the patient to that provided by a CMHT (rarely more than 1–2 contacts per month), and demonstrated that the patient can cope with this without relapse. Joint visits with the new keyworker are usual.

'A positive step'

It is important that the handover is construed in terms of the patient's progress – not that they no longer 'justify' the AO team input any more. This would be experienced as rejection by the patient and condescension by the receiving team. It is also important to accept that a relapse is more likely at times of handover no matter how skilfully handled. A willingness to acknowledge this helps smooth relationships all round. Sometimes a mistake may have been made and the patient may need to come back to the AO team.

Team days and development

All teams need to take time out to reflect and monitor where they are going if they are not to drift and become stale (Chapter 2). This process is probably even more important for assertive outreach teams than many others because of the level of disability and chronicity of most of the patients. With a group of patients in which changes are likely to be slow and for whom connections with the wider society are limited it is all too easy to lose track of realistic ambitions and adopt an unacceptably dependent relationship. As in older mental hospitals AO staff work hard to help patients stabilize their lives and recover from their illnesses. Not surprisingly they may have difficulty in recognizing when that improved functioning reflects recovery rather than the result of, and the need for, their continuing clinical input. Just as highly structured reviews have been stressed for this form of team so team away-days and reviews of the operational policy are enormously important.

The slow turnover in such a team threatens to foster complacency and lack of clinical ambition. All that has been written about the need for regular development meetings and honest self examination in away-days for general teams needs to be underlined for assertive outreach teams.

Conclusions

Assertive outreach teams are probably the most established of the proposed specialized teams and undoubtedly the most firmly based on research. How they relate to other components of an integrated mental health service will vary, as will their professional composition and responsibilities. Variation in assertive outreach teams should be less given this longer experience and accumulated evidence. However, it is clear from an examination of those established in London (Wright *et al.* 2003) that there are marked variations in practice. Their value in the care of revolving door psychotic patients is overwhelming. Ignoring the evidence for the role of integrated medical staff in the teams, or ignoring an emphasis on medication management cannot easily be justified.

Despite variation in the application of the acknowledged principles of Assertive Outreach the core approach is clear. Although these principles are well recognized they are not without significant difficulties and uncertainties in how best to apply them. There are internal tensions in the model that have to be worked with – the tension between model fidelity and individualization of care, the conflict between the duty of care (often manifest in 'assertiveness') and individual patient civil rights, the respect and support for autonomy and the occasional need for compulsory treatment. Assertive outreach teams benefit by having a well-articulated theory and practice guidelines but this brings the risk of premature institutionalization. They need to maintain a broad psychosocial approach to their patients while not losing sight of the central importance of evidence based medical practice. In short their research based and prescribed approach is both their greatest strength and their Achilles' heel.

CHAPTER 5

Early intervention teams

Origins of early intervention teams

The onset of psychoses

For several decades psychotic illnesses have been understood mainly as episodes of positive symptoms, followed by full or partial recovery for variable periods. In schizophrenia this recovery was often associated with disabilities and the development of negative symptoms. The first contact with mental health services followed from the patient's first 'breakdown'. Functioning prior to the breakdown was recognized as important – for instance in schizophrenia the existence of a premorbid 'schizoid personality' (withdrawn, shy, aloof, a bit odd) implied a poorer outcome. This impact on outcome was understood either as the interaction of the illness with the individual's coping resources, or that these personality traits were markers for a more severe form of disease. Whichever view was taken 'premorbid' functioning was seen as just that – *premorbid*, not a part of the disorder.

Cracks have appeared in this view. Cohort studies following up children from birth into their thirties have convincingly shown that those who go on to develop schizophrenia in adult life have significant difficulties even before adolescence (Done *et al.* 1994, Jones *et al.* 1994). Some even experienced psychosis-like symptoms as early as at the age of 11 (Poulton *et al.* 2000). In short there has been a re-evaluation of schizophrenia to a more pervasive neurodevelopmental disorder – a return to a view more like Kraepelin's when he first described dementia praecox (Kraepelin 1919).

The temporal relationship between positive and negative symptoms has also come under review. Comprehensive structured assessments of schizophrenia in research studies have revealed that negative symptoms are often present right at the start of the illness (Fenton and McGlashan 1994) – it is just that the clinician's attention is usually focused then on the more dramatic and distressing positive ones.

Duration of untreated psychosis (DUP)

Several recent pathways to care studies (how patients came to obtain treatment and care) have shown that patients had often been ill and deteriorating for several months before they sought treatment. The association of an 'insidious' onset with poorer outcomes is now often interpreted more as the longer a patient goes undiagnosed and untreated with early schizophrenia, the worse they do. It has been proposed that periods

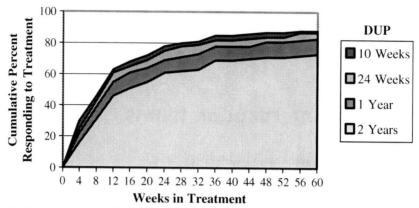

Fig. 5.1 Time to remission by prior duration of psychosis (after Lieberman 1996).

of active psychosis are 'toxic' for the brain, entrenching dysfunctional mechanisms. The longer the patient is actively ill the more damage is done to mental functioning, often irreversibly so. One strong piece of evidence for this belief is the association between DUP and time to recovery in first episode disorders (Lieberman *et al.* 1996). As demonstrated in Fig. 5.1 the time to recovery in their study is considerably shorter for first episode patients treated earlier in their illness.

Is DUP really 'toxic'?

While there is support for this belief that DUP has a direct influence on outcome there are still some doubts. Craig and colleagues (Craig *et al.* 2000) failed to find any association between DUP and outcome at 2 years. Similarly Barnes and colleagues (Barnes *et al.* 2000) failed to find the association to be 'independent' (i.e. while a longer DUP was strongly associated with poor outcome it was also associated with other features predicting a poor outcome). When these features were controlled for there was no association of outcome remaining with DUP. The features that were independently associated with poor outcome in their study were those of insidious onset, poor social functioning (e.g. dropped out of college, not working, isolated etc.) all of which would result in later *detection* of the illness.

Long-term outcome of schizophrenia

Perhaps even more sobering is a comparison of long-term outcome studies of schizophrenia over the course of the last century. Hegarty's review (Hegarty *et al.* 1994) contains studies from before there were any antipsychotics at all – so patients effectively had a lifetime of DUP. The absence of any major difference in the long-term outcome of the disease over this 100 years must question the concept of 'toxicity' of DUP. This is not to say, however, that treatment makes no difference. Far from it – it is clear that reducing the severity and duration of each psychotic episode is immensely important for each individual patient. However if DUP had a specific and powerful effect on the course of the illness then the long-term outcome should be very significantly better in later studies, but it is not. So caution is indicated.

Prodromal psychoses and the 'critical period'

Prodromes and high risk individuals

The real impetus for early intervention services has come from the work of Pat McGorry and colleagues in Australia (McGorry and Jackson 1999) and Max Birchwood in the UK (Birchwood *et al.* 1997). They have focused on prodromal psychotic episodes and high risk groups which appear strongly predictive of subsequent schizophrenia. McGorry studied treatment with antipsychotics in high risk patients with strong family histories who demonstrated specific abnormalities (usually '*BLIPS*' – Brief Limited Psychotic Symptoms, or severe social withdrawal and poor school functioning). Interventions with prodromal episodes and high risk groups is described in greater detail below ('High-risk and Prodromal Intervention').

The critical period

As a psychologist Birchwood emphasizes the consequences to the young adult of the onset of a psychotic illness just when they are forming their identity and establishing themselves in the world. This early period of illness is when much social competence and functioning can be lost ('The critical period hypothesis' (Birchwood *et al.* 1998)). This is an alternative understanding of DUP stressing social and developmental vulnerability rather than neural toxicity. The 'social decline' observed in schizophrenia is maximal either just before the first episode or at that first episode, rather than from the cumulative effects of repeated relapses. Equally importantly the risk of life threatening crises due to aggression or suicide are highest in the early stages of the disorder (two-thirds occurring in the first 5 years). Outcome at 2 years also predicts that at 13 years (Loebel *et al.* 1992).

Overall the case for ensuring that high quality comprehensive services are focused on young victims of psychosis is overwhelming. Not only does the science point towards it, but there are ethical and practical reasons for intervening early. Simple humanity demands we reduce the duration of psychosis because these disorders are so distressing. We know from studies of established psychoses that patients who have the support of families do better and that losing contact with families is a common consequence of the first breakdown. Providing comprehensive and generous support for the family at this time meets carers' legitimate needs and also fosters coping skills, which may help the family stay together.

Louise, a 23-year-old woman, was referred to the early intervention service following a crisis admission to an adult ward with a three-year history of hallucinations, passivity experiences, persecutory delusions, mood swings, social withdrawal, and recurrent conflicts with her mother, usually under the influence of alcohol. Her mother had repeatedly sought the GP's advice but Louise had refused to see him. Following a crisis presentation to the A&E, she was referred to the CMHT and seen by the team social worker. Her problems were attributed to family dynamics and she was provided information on local anger management courses. At the mother's insistence, the GP made another referral requesting a medical review and the consultant psychiatrist saw her. She was thought to be exhibiting 'possible prodromal symptoms of psychosis' and community follow-up was suggested. She defaulted from follow-up and the team discharged her from their care. Six months later she was admitted after a serious self-harm attempt and psychotic symptoms were elicited during the inpatient stay. Despite intensive input by the early intervention service over a two-year period, she stayed significantly disabled with negative symptoms and transferred to the ACT team.

Variety of early intervention teams

Early Intervention Service (EIS) teams demonstrate much greater variety than other specialist teams. They differ markedly in both structure and function – including what they emphasize, who they serve and what treatments they offer (Edwards *et al.* 2000). This range derives from two main sources – first the tension between functional specialization and locality focus, and second the research interests of the local clinical leaders.

Specialism versus locality focus

This is a tension inherent in the remit of EIS teams – they are meant to be highly specialized and yet locally based and 'holistic' in approach. Narrowing the clinical focus will inevitably increase the catchment area required to provide the patient group. For example a generic CMHT quickly acquires a caseload of 2–300 from a population of 30,000–40,000 whereas an assertive outreach team focusing on difficult revolving door psychotic patients would serve a population of 200,000 to fill a caseload of 100. The NHS Plan suggests one first onset service per million population. Clearly this could not work effectively as a single team. The caseload size would be excessive and there would be no possibility of building up local knowledge or relationships. Intensity and comprehensiveness of treatment, community-focus, and the target population are therefore three elements which inevitably interact to drive the varied configurations of early intervention teams. The current recommendation is 3–4 teams in each service for one million population.

Research interests

The high profile EIS teams which preceded the UK policy initiative evolved from local research interests. Birchwood's research interests in psychosocial interventions and CBT characterizes the teams in Birmingham. McGorry's focus on prodromes and high risk patients in Melbourne or McFarlane's family interventions in the US have each produced clinical cultures and practices that are highly distinct.

These scientific differences play themselves out in quite basic issues. One team emphasizes the specificity of interventions and therefore insists on careful diagnosis and a restriction to patients with schizophrenia. Another emphasizes the personal and social impact of psychosis and essentially ignores diagnosis but focuses on stigma, work, and education. Not surprisingly such teams will differ in the catchment area size, the staff composition of the team, and even the age served. A consequence is that the description of EIS teams in this chapter will invariably involve a range of practices. Time will tell which configurations are more durable and which interventions provide most benefit.

NIMHE expert briefing

The National Institute for Mental Health in England (NIMHE) has produced a series of expert briefings and that for EIS teams was published in the summer of 2003 (NIMHE 2003). This short document includes a summary of the essential elements of an Early Intervention Service as agreed by 21 expert clinicians using a 'Delphi process'. This is a recognized technique for promoting and measuring concensus about complex issues. The following table outlines these elements. While the document points out that there is broad agreement between these clinicians and the more detailed Policy Implementation Guide, it is characterized by a less prescriptive approach. Many of these essential elements will be explored further here with the aim of making them more concrete.

Essential elements of an Early Intervention Service (EIS) (NIMHE 2003)	
Focus of Intervention	**Element**
Client group	• EIS should deal with people in their first episode of psychosis
Team structure	EIS should: • be composed of staff whose sole or main responsibility is to the EIS • have at least one member trained in CBT • incorporate medical, social, and psychological models • emphasize clients' views on their problems and level of functioning
Team membership	EIS should: • include a consultant psychiatrist with dedicated sessions • include at least one psychiatric nurse • include a clinical psychologist • have support from Child and Adolescent Mental Health Services (CAMHS) when prescribing for under 16-year-olds • Have close links with CAMHS Note: There was also good consensus for inclusion of: social worker, an occupational therapist, and a support worker

(continued)

Essential elements of an Early Intervention Service (EIS) (NIMHE 2003) *(continued)*

Focus of Intervention	Element

Initial assessment   EIS should:

- assess clients referred on suspicion rather than certainty of psychosis
- encourage direct referrals from primary care
- have access to translation services
- not be concerned about precise diagnosis so long as in psychotic spectrum
- offer a rapid initial assessment
- regularly audit effectiveness of referral pathways and training programmes
- accept referrals from Child and Adolescent Mental Health Services
- identify areas of distress

An EIS assessment should include:

- a psychiatric history and mental state examination
- a social functioning and resource assessment
- an assessment of risk (including suicide)
- an assessment of the client's family
- the client's aspirations and understanding of their illness
- an EIS assessment should be multi-disciplinary
- each EIS client should have a relapse risk assessment
- the goal of early contact should be engagement rather than treatment

Engagement   EIS should:

- have an assertive approach to engaging the client and their family/ social network
- not close the case if client fails to engage
- allocate a key worker to all clients accepted into the service
- provide services away from traditional psychiatric settings to avoid stigma

Non-drug treatment   EIS should:

- emphasize identification and treatment of depression among clients
- emphasize identification and treatment of suicidal thinking
- provide CBT to clients with treatment-resistant positive symptoms
- provide clients with educational materials about psychosis
- Each EIS client should have a relapse prevention plan

Drug treatment

- EIS should use low-dose atypical neuroleptics as the first-line drug treatment
- Clients with disabling negative symptoms should have review of drug treatment
- EIS should actively involve clients in decisions about medication
- EIS clients should receive detailed information about medication

(continued)

Essential elements of an Early Intervention Service (EIS) (NIMHE 2003) *(continued)*

Focus of Intervention	Element
Relatives and significant others	EIS should: • engage a client's family/significant others at an early stage • involve family and significant others in client's ongoing review process • provide families with psychoeducation and support • provide families with Psychoeducational Family Intervention • A relapse prevention plan should be shared with the client's family/ significant others
Admission to hospital	• EIS should have access to separate age-appropriate inpatient facilities for young people • EIS should be able to provide intensive community support when a client is in crisis • Each EIS service user/family/carer should know how to access support in a crisis • EIS clients should be able to access out-of-hours support from a 24-hour crisis team • When a client is an inpatient, EIS team should be actively involved in inpatient reviews • When a client is an inpatient, EIS team should be actively involved in discharge planning • EIS should be prepared to use its powers under mental health legislation
Community connections	• There should be a single point of contact so primary care and other agencies can check out potential concerns/resources and ease the confusion of roles/responsibilities

Who is it for?

This is not as straightforward as it might seem. In some parts of Australia there has been a radical restructuring of the boundary between adult mental health services and CAMHS (Child and Adolescent Mental Health Services) with the development of 'youth' services. These serve all mental health problems, psychosis included, for an age range of 12–25 years. This restructuring derived from local concerns and will be watched with interest. In North American and European EIS teams there is a wide range of upper age limits from 26–45 years.

In the UK, however, EIS teams are explicitly for young individuals with psychotic illnesses. As outlined above there are different views about whether or not this should be all psychotic illnesses or just schizophrenia, only first breakdowns or any relapse and what the age limits and the duration of contact should be. Given that the UK mental health services are charged with establishing 50 such services over the next 3 years these questions will have to be resolved locally before there is consensus. Different services will undoubtedly adopt different approaches. These will be strategic judgements – there simply is no research evidence on which to base them. The relative merits of several decisions conflict with each other.

All psychoses or just schizophrenia?

The presentation of a first episode of psychosis is often a confusing and dramatic one. Patients are frequently disturbed and agitated with a broad mixture of symptoms such that a firm diagnosis is not obvious. Distinguishing with certainty between schizophrenia, a manic episode or even a drug-induced state may be impossible for some time in many cases. However, once schizophrenia has been identified there is considerable diagnostic stability.

The UK Policy Implementation Guide (PIG) recommends that services should have '… an emphasis on managing symptoms rather than diagnosis'. For this reason a number of teams (e.g. The Lambeth Early Onset Team, LEO (Garety et al. 1997)) take all psychotic patients and consider preoccupations with differential diagnosis to be distracting and unhelpful. Their focus is on the disruption that psychosis causes to young people. On the other hand the North Birmingham team (IRIS – Initiative to Reduce Impact of Schizophrenia) has developed its services specifically for individuals with schizophrenia although they 'keep the goal posts wide' (MacMillan and Shiers 2000). IRIS hands on patients if their illness subsequently becomes obvious as Bipolar Affective Disorder or drug induced. Their rationale is that the range of interventions in which they are skilled are developed for schizophrenia.

IRIS core principles include (MacMillan and Shiers 2000)

- A youth and user focus.
- The importance of early and assertive engagement.
- The embracing of diagnostic uncertainty.
- Treatment to be provided in the least restrictive and stigmatizing setting.
- An emphasis on social roles.
- A family orientated approach.

Specificity of psychosocial interventions

Research evidence for the interventions which these teams emphasize (see below 'specific skills and interventions') hardly supports an exclusive focus on schizophrenia. For various practical reasons most psychosocial interventions for psychotic illnesses are initially developed with schizophrenia patients. This research bias towards schizophrenia is widespread and may simply reflect that schizophrenia patients are easier to enrol in research studies than others such as bipolar patients (Clement et al. 2003). They also have more enduring symptoms so that efficacy can be judged.

Several psychosocial interventions (such as behavioural family management to reduce high EE) are effective beyond schizophrenia. Motivational interviewing was developed with substance abuse disorders (Rollinick *et al.* 1992) but is equally effective for improving medication compliance in a range of psychotic patients (Kemp *et al.* 1998). Relapse signature training and intervention has been most effectively demonstrated in bipolar disorder (Perry *et al.* 1999). On the other hand, no studies of a specific psychosocial intervention which is successful with schizophrenia have shown them to be *ineffective* with other psychotic disorders. The relative non-specificity of these interventions gives little support for restricting by diagnosis.

Schizophrenia patients are more likely to be offered vocational rehabilitation because of their obvious profound interpersonal disabilities and deficit states. However, unemployment and educational disruption are probably just as common in mania and drug induced psychoses. Disruptions in these latter groups may be more amenable to prompt intervention and some argue that, while not so obviously handicapped, there is more to gain by intervention with them.

Resources and work-load

A more convincing argument for restricting EIS teams to schizophrenia probably derives from resource and capacity issues. Inner city settings services for a one million population would comprise 3–4 teams each of which can expect upwards of 150 new cases of schizophrenia a year (Singh *et al.* 2002). Depending on how long the team keeps the patients (see the next section) this will fully stretch, or indeed overstretch, their capacity. If there is simply not enough resource to take on all new psychosis patients a diagnostic filter is one pragmatic solution.

The pattern of work also may favour restricting the team to schizophrenia patients. Young bipolar patients are particularly disruptive and much of their early care may involve repeated hospitalizations. Where teams take responsibility for inpatient care (see below) these patients with more episodic disorders can monopolize their resources and prevent the development of psychosocial programmes.

A first-episode service or a youth service?

Early intervention teams need to decide whether they will restrict themselves to an age range or to patients experiencing their first breakdown. The UK Policy Implementation Guide (Department of Health 2001) stipulates 'Patients between the ages of 14 and 35 with a first presentation of psychotic symptoms.'

Effectively this is giving priority to age. Almost half of first psychotic episodes (especially in women) are over the age of 35 years. Most services currently being established operate an age cut off around 30 years acknowledging an emphasis on a 'youth service'. Many staff who work in these services consider that the 'youth orientation' is what marks them out rather than the profile of specific interventions. It emphasizes a tolerant, somewhat anti-establishment air that appeals to adolescents and young adults.

While treating an individual thought to have a first episode, it is not unusual to find that they have had a previous psychosis, either untreated or treated elsewhere. It may not be until rapport has been established, or they are recovered enough to give their history fully, that this is discovered. Having taken on patients few services would discharge them simply because of such a history, although some do.

Lower age of acceptance

The lower age of acceptance remains controversial. The difficulty for the rare individual who develops a psychotic illness in early adolescence is that they do not fit easily into *any* service. It is important to remember just how rare such very early onsets are. The misconception that schizophrenia is a disease of adolescence is very persistent. Indeed the PIG repeats this misunderstanding by quoting the mean age of onset at 22 years when in fact the mean is 27 years for men and 31 for women (Hafner *et al.* 1994). A second peak of onset for women is between 45–54 years (Castle and Murray 1993; Hafner *et al.* 1991) – well above the cut off for such teams as currently proposed.

In short, schizophrenia is *not* a disorder of adolescence (although problems in adolescence are very common before frank psychosis). Early onset cases (e.g. aged 18–20) consider themselves adults and would normally be cared for by adult teams. Cases below age 18 are comparatively rare and, when very ill, are also generally cared for by adult teams because they know about psychosis whereas few Child and Adolescent teams are equipped to cope.

It would be misleading to suggest that there is consensus on how to manage the rare cases of very early onset (e.g. the 4.4% of presentations aged under 16 years (Singh *et al.* 2002)). From age 16 up most professionals anticipate that the new teams will be the most appropriate service but there really is not enough experience about the very young. It is highly likely that they will be dealt with on a case-by-case basis until a consensus evolves.

Duration of follow-up with the team

Early intervention teams are described as being based on the assertive outreach model (Chapter 4) although some of their practices (e.g. 'zoning' see below) clearly are not typically AO. The AO approach involves a commitment to regular, close follow-up even during periods of relative recovery. The approach is flexible in its day-to-day application with efforts made to remain in contact with patients for several years. The advantages of this include being able to work with the patient and family on issues such as social and vocational recovery and coping skills etc., when the clinical picture is not dominated by positive symptoms and managing crises.

How long this commitment should be is still being explored. The PIG suggests 3 years and this approach is used in North Birmingham, whereas LEO aims to hold on to patients for up to 5 years. The EPPIC service in Melbourne has a follow-up of only 18 months. These longer durations will be hard to sustain in busy teams and the consensus figure, when it does arise, will probably be determined as much by capacity as science. Certainly the current clinical ambitions of such teams require at least 2–3 years to achieve.

Flexibility over longer duration

As with all services these figures are guidelines, not absolute rules. Some patients will just be settling, fully engaged, and be in a highly productive collaboration with the team at 3 years. Obviously it would be foolish to discharge them then. Similarly some patients may have made a rapid recovery and want to be discharged well before the 3 years are up. An example presented in one service was of a young man who had suffered a classical schizophrenic breakdown but recovered very well within 9 months and had gone on to university. He was very keen to sever his contact with the team who were equally anxious to keep him on their books. There is a clear conflict between the team's and the patient's wishes. These ethical dilemmas are not unusual in assertive outreach teams generally. They will require especially careful attention in EIS teams where patients are still developing their identity and have not necessarily accepted that of an individual with an enduring disorder.

Problems with handing back to routine services

A specialist team needs boundaries to establish a distinct identity for its specialization. Although the EIS is blessed with clarity about the time for patients to move on (either time with the team, or age) in practice this is a vexed issue. Good teams have high morale with members proud of what they do and convinced of its value, and this will have transmitted itself to the patient and family. A consequence is that transfer out can easily feel like a rejection. This is dealt with in some depth for AO teams in Chapter 4, but is even more difficult in EIS teams. Not only is the EIS team likely to be better resourced than either the AOT or CMHT the patient moves on to, but this moving on often implies a sense of the '*long term*' that may have, up till now, been avoided. It may also involve a shift to a more medical, less broadly psychosocial, approach.

As outlined in Chapter 4 it is essential to find ways to frame the move in terms of '*progress*' and '*moving on*' rather than of '*having come to the end of your time*'. The move to more mainstream services needs to be worked on as a goal of treatment, often over several months. This should involve genuine joint working with the receiving team – not simply a handover of responsibility with the care plan unchanged. The treatment goals should be negotiated with the patient and carers jointly between EIS and the new keyworker.

Team components

EIS teams are more confusing to understand than other specialist teams because differing interests in the model teams have resulted in quite different structures and functions. These can be combined with different priorities assigned to them or they may even be dealt with in specific sub-teams. For simplicity the three major components of the potential service will be described as individual teams although most services will combine the functions within one team.

EIS team components

- Continuing care team (AO team).
- Early detection team.
- Prodromal treatment team.

Continuing care or community team (The assertive outreach team)

Focus on engagement

All EIS services will have a multidisciplinary team which is broadly based on the assertive outreach model (Chapter 4). This offers continuing multidisciplinary treatment and follow-up that is individually assessed, needs-based, and comprehensive in content. The approach is assertive and non-institutional with an emphasis on meeting the patient in their own environment and trying to solve the problems that arise there. EIS teams place a high priority on engagement – traumatic first admissions and young people's wishes to deny the severity of their illnesses can make it very difficult to establish a working relationship. Typically EIS teams, like AO teams, are prepared to be patient building a strong alliance before pushing treatment.

Wayne is a 19-year-old man of African-Caribbean origin who disengaged from the CMHT following a rapid symptomatic recovery from a first-episode psychosis. His initial contact with services had been through a very traumatic admission involving the police. He stopped medication after discharge. Although not thought to be detainable, concerns remained about his mental state. He agreed to see the early intervention team who spent several initial weekly sessions helping him resolve his accommodation and financial problems. During these sessions, he gradually started discussing the events leading up to his admission and began accepting that he might have been ill. His refusal to re-start medication was not allowed to jeopardise the engagement process. At regular intervals, the keyworker discussed the risk of relapse and early warning signs with him. During his re-housing, his psychotic symptoms began to emerge and were monitored by increasing the key worker contact to twice a week. As his anxiety mounted, he agreed to re-try low-dose antipsychotics. His symptoms resolved quickly and he agreed to continue medication. He has successfully returned to education and remained symptoms free and medication compliant for a further 18 months.

A particular aim is to protect social and educational functioning. Following AO principles the team has a fixed caseload, both overall and for each individual case manager. Handover and shift arrangements are similar to AO teams with 7-day working being established in most, but there are variations between teams in shifts and extended hours working.

Referrals usually come from CMHTs (although, unlike AO Teams, direct GP referral may be encouraged). Details of new referrals are often recorded in structured referral forms such as Fig. 5.2. The value of such referral forms is discussed in Chapter 2. At the

Early Intervention Service Client Referral Form	
Date of referral: _____	Referral received by: _____
Date ref received: _____	Referring Agent/Team: _____
	YES/NO
Is individual aware of referral to Early Intervention:	YES/NO

Personal Details:

Client Name: _____	Unit No: _____
Address: _____	Tel No: _____
_____	Title: _____
_____	Gender: _____
Date of Birth: _____	Ethnic Origin: _____
Marital Status: _____	Language spoken: _____
Other Agencies Involved: _____	Interpreter needed: YES/NO

GP Address: _____	Current RMO: _____
_____	Next of Kin: _____
_____	(Relationship) _____
_____	Address: _____
Tel No: _____	_____
	Tel No: _____

Please give a brief personal/social and mental health history, including:

Living circumstances: Alone ☐ Family ☐ Sheltered ☐
Previous contact with psychiatric services: YES/NO
If yes, reason:
No of months/years of contact:
Employment: Full time ☐ Part time ☐ Unemployed ☐
Details of education, inc age left school, qualifications etc:

Any physical problems, please detail:
....
Reasons for referral:
....
Current medication:
....
Use of illicit substances (if any, please list)

Any history of self harm/suicide attempts/harm to others (please detail):
....
Forensic History (if any, please detail any current/pending Court proceedings, probation orders etc):

FOR EARLY INTERVENTION USE ONLY:

Contact made to referring agent on: _____
Outcome: ACCEPTED/NOT ACCEPTED
Reasons: _____
Allocated to: _____
Form filled out by: _____

Fig. 5.2 EIS referral form

very least they identify whether patients meet the team's remit or not, and they are invaluable in audit and defining local relationships. Common patterns of referrals taken on compared to those not taken on for treatment can be identified from them thereby improving local understanding of the service.

The composition of the continuing care team is broadly similar to that described for AO Teams in Chapter 4 except that there are usually specific individuals responsible for vocational support and for dealing with substance abuse. There are three important ways, however, in which the EIS AO team differs from the 'standard' AO model.

Duration of follow-up

While Stein and Test (Stein and Test 1980) proposed a 'no discharge policy' for their original team most AO teams decide clinically when patients are ready to move on. Usually this is when the clinical picture has settled and when the individual has been stabilized over an extended period (see Chapter 4). EIS teams, however, have explicit policies about discharge which are based on ideology and resources as described earlier. While these vary from team to team (e.g. the PIG recommends 3 years, LEO aims for 5 years) what is characteristic is that the time is definite and explicit. While this can occasionally be overridden for clinical reasons it remains a fundamental variation from AO practice.

Zoning and caseloads

Few EIS services have small caseloads. Indeed most have caseloads equivalent to 30 per case manager – more like CMHTs than AO teams. These large caseloads reflect their follow-up policy with patients kept on the books for long periods when they may be asymptomatic and, even, fully recovered. These patients are kept on what is, effectively, outpatient monitoring (e.g. monthly contact or less to check things are okay). To ensure that patients are able to receive comprehensive AO-like care when they are unwell the team explicitly divides its caseload into 'zones' reflecting level of needs.

Traffic light system

A traffic light system is used for simplicity. '*Red*' zone patients are those requiring the full ACT approach. These patients are judged to be on the brink of relapse and admission if they do not receive comprehensive and intensive care. They have visits that are more than weekly and they are mentioned by name at every handover and generally receive the full range of active multidisciplinary input. '*Amber*' patients are those who are not currently judged to be at imminent risk of relapse but still require complex interventions and support. For instance they may be working very actively with the substance abuse specialist or with the vocational specialist to get back into college. '*Green*' patients are those who are stable and getting on with their lives and receiving only intermittent monitoring. Where teams rely heavily on a 'white board' to manage their work load this is usually broken down by key worker and within each key worker area further divided by zone.

Zoning

Red: Imminent risk of relapse. Full 'ACT' treatment. Contact > 1 per week. Named each handover.

Amber: Not at imminent risk of relapse but receiving substantive ongoing treatment.

Green: Stable. Receiving only outpatient monitoring.

Benefits policy

AO teams usually aim to obtain the maximum social welfare benefits for their patients. This is to improve their quality of life, as an aspect of advocacy, and also as a very effective tool for engagement. The situation is not so simple in EIS teams where the 'benefit trap' can be particularly destructive. EIS teams are highly committed to getting their patients rapidly back into work or education wherever possible. It would also be counter-productive, so early in the illness, to be pessimistic about their capacity for recovery. EIS services are much more cautious about reducing the financial incentives to either starting or returning to work. Too much is at stake.

There are important differences between the two types of teams in the balance of training and encouragement to develop versus the need to support and prevent deterioration. The latter are significantly more prominent in AO teams for individuals with several years of SMI. EIS teams probably 'push' their patients more. Being circumspect about obtaining too much early financial security is one way of encouraging growth. Obviously these decisions require considerable sensitivity.

Early detection teams

All EIS teams aim to reduce DUP by shortening the time from first recognizing that something is amiss to obtaining assessment and treatment. As teams gain experience and confidence in establishing the diagnosis and introducing comprehensive treatments, delays will inevitably reduce. Some services, however, go beyond this. They set up either a small separate team or a sub-team to raise awareness of psychosis ('raising the index of suspicion') so that 'recognizing that something is amiss' will occur earlier. This early detection team will have an educational function – training local GPs and their staff about warning signs of psychosis, giving talks in schools and colleges about how to recognize when withdrawal or odd behaviour may be more than just adolescent turmoil.

An important aspect of this educational role is to try and reduce the stigma attached to mental illness through increased public awareness. An easily obtained, relatively informal assessment process serves the dual function of reducing stigma and increasing access. The early detection team will deliberately encourage a low threshold for consultation and referral. Assessments will often be in GP surgeries or other non 'mental health' facilities. If the 'clinic' is genuinely non-stigmatizing then assessing healthy individuals does no harm and there is much to gain by early detection.

High-risk and prodromal teams

Some EISs go beyond early detection of psychosis and try to intervene in high-risk groups even before frank psychosis. This is a controversial area and generally restricted to research-based teams but can cause confusion in understanding EIS teams. Most of the work has been done in Melbourne by Pat McGorry and his EPPIC (Early Psychosis Prevention and Intervention Centre) team (McGorry *et al.* 1996) and both the best known UK teams have established such services. LEO has its OASIS (Outreach and Support in South London) team in South London and North Birmingham (Birchwood *et al.* 2000) has its EDIT (Early Detection and Treatment) team. Both work on the understanding that there are individuals who are identifiable as being at high risk of developing a psychotic illness.

Psychotic prodromes

These high-risk individuals are often thought to demonstrate a psychotic 'prodrome'. This is a characteristic picture that is not, in itself, psychosis, but a stage in the *development* of the psychosis. It is a process (not a risk factor) that indicates that a psychotic breakdown is on the way. There is controversy about whether there really are prodromes for psychoses, what is the 'transition' point and how can they be distinguished from the early emergence of the psychosis.

There are now several studies showing that giving low dose antipsychotic medication to individuals with 'early warning signs' reduces 'transition' to psychosis (Gaebel *et al.* 1993; Marder *et al.* 1984, 1994). These were small, open studies.

Identifying high-risk subjects

Current teams follow the same general principles in identifying 'ultra high-risk' individuals developed by McGorry. This is a much more tightly defined target population than the high risk groups traditionally identified solely by genetics. This criteria for identification are:

Criteria for ultra high-risk subjects

A. 1. Family history of psychosis in first degree relative, and

   2. non-specific symptoms and functioning producing a reduction in GAF of over 30 points in the last 12 months,

or

B.   attenuated positive schizophrenia symptoms >1 week but sub threshold in intensity for DSM-IV diagnosis,

or

C.   brief episodes of positive schizophrenia symptoms (BLIPS) <1 week but reaching threshold in intensity for DSM-IV diagnosis.

Impact of intervention

McGorry and his team in Melbourne (McGorry *et al.* 2002) have shown that intervening in this group with low dose risperidone and CBT significantly reduces the rate of progression to full psychosis. It remains unclear from this study whether this is a preventative effect or simply delays onset. Larger and more rigorous studies are needed to determine that. This study had only 30 subjects in each group and could not be 'blinded' – raters, patients, and staff knew what the treatment was. What is remarkable from this study, however, is that *all* the experimental subjects were functioning better at 12 months. Concerns that 'labelling' these young patients might damage them were not confirmed.

This aspect of EIS has been dealt with at some length – out of proportion to its clinical profile – because it is easily confused with relapse prevention (see below) or early detection and it poses enormous ethical dilemmas. When establishing an EIS there needs to be clarity about whether or not treating high risk individuals is going to be part of the service. On current evidence it would be hard to justify in routine practice. Clarity is needed to distinguish these procedures and terms must not be used sloppily. This table summarizes the main differences between these component teams.

Elements of Early Intervention Teams

	Early Detection Team	Prodromal Intervention Team	Continuing Care (AO) Team
Age Range	12–30	14–35	14–35
First episode of psychosis	✔	✔	✔
Early detection	✔	✔	Some
Prodromal intervention	Possibly	✔	No
Psychosocial intervention	✔	Varies	✔
'A youth service'	✔	✔	Some
Population served	Unclear/large	Unclear/large	200,000–350,000
Location of treatment	Home/neighbourhood/ clinic	Clinic	Home/neighbourhood
Duration of treatment	Screen for PI or CC team	1–2 years	2–5 years
Diagnostic focus	Symptoms	Prodrome	Psychosis or schizophrenia
AO approach	No	No	✔
Zoning	No	No	✔
Vocational rehab/ social inclusion focus	✔	No	✔

Specific EIS interventions

EIS teams are more likely than others to define themselves in terms of what specific treatments they provide. Although virtually all of these treatments will be found in other specialist teams (apart from high-risk and prodrome treatments) they have a greater prominence in EIS teams. For instance family support and treatments are part of any high quality comprehensive service but dominate in EIS services for fairly obvious reasons. Not only do these core interventions comprise a greater proportion of the working week in EIS teams but they have also been refined and operationalized more thoroughly. Dealing with them here does not imply, however, that their place is restricted to EIS teams.

Family support

Family interventions for individuals with psychotic illnesses are broadly divided into three categories: illness education (often called psychoeducation), ongoing support (usually in local groups but often individually at times of crisis), and lastly, for those who need it, formal problem solving interventions to reduce emotional arousal.

Family interventions

- Illness education (psychoeducation).
- Support groups.
- Behaviour family management.

Illness education

The importance of ensuring that both patients and their families understand the nature of the illness and the purpose (and side-effects) of their treatments has become increasingly obvious. In long-term disorders it is unrealistic to rely on professionals alone to 'manage' the illness for the patient. Time and again it has been demonstrated that family members may misinterpret features of the illness in moral or behavioural terms (e.g. viewing negative symptoms in schizophrenia as laziness, or failing to realize that their son is preoccupied with hallucinations and not simply ignoring them).

Without an understanding of the medicines, families (and friends) may misinterpret early side-effects such as sedation or tremor as symptomatic worsening and encourage the patient to stop them. Many families are worried that all psychotropic drugs are habit forming (like diazepam) and may fear that this will complicate the patient's problems further. With increasing understanding of the illness families can support the patient and also help the staff in tailoring treatments.

Confronting fear

Simply understanding what is going on can also reduce anxiety. Doctors and nurses often worry that informing the family about the seriousness of the illness and the side-effects of the treatments will frighten them off. Experience teaches otherwise. Families and patients often think the worst, and although the open acknowledgement of the seriousness can be stressful, most welcome greater knowledge. While it may not 'reassure' them, it does reduce uncertainty and helps them marshal their emotional resources. Giving a diagnosis can also help – it establishes the problem as a medical illness which is being treated by specialists. Discussing side-effects of medication, for instance, does not result in poorer compliance but quite the contrary (Chaplin and Kent 1998). In many ways this should not surprise us – families and patients have first hand experience of the illness and treatment. We are rarely telling them anything new (Kosky and Burns 1995), but helping them construct a framework within which to cope.

Engagement

Family and patient education has been increasingly recognized as a valuable stage in engagement. It provides a safe space in which to get to know each other better and carries a powerful message about respect and collaboration. Time spent explaining the issues shows that one takes the family seriously – both their distress but also their capacity to make a difference. It will often be in stark contrast to experiences in some other branches of medicine where they will simply have been told what to do.

Even simple interchanges help. For example, if one does not know the answer to a question (e.g. 'What is the upper dose range of this new drug?') but agrees to find it out and report back next time, this can be very positive. It models honest acknowledgement of the level of expertise that we have, it demonstrates a willingness to share this and, when the answer is provided at the next appointment, a real commitment to carrying through.

It is sobering to remember that the vast bulk of complaints against doctors and nurses in all branches of medicine are not about the quality of care but their failure to explain it. We are assessed on how we communicate more than on the effectiveness of our treatments. Families and patients who feel heard, understood, and treated with respect will trust staff and work with them against the illness.

Printed material and videos

Taking in emotionally laden information is difficult and we know that patients retain only a tiny proportion of what they are told at consultations. Illness education requires repetition and reinforcement. Increasingly there are high quality publications (both leaflets and books and also now videos) that can be given to families to supplement face-to-face education. These materials are, however, *only supplements*. They are not an adequate alternative to discussing directly the individual patient and *their* illness and *their* treatment. Their value is that the patient and family can study them at length and ask questions and gain clarification when you next meet.

'A shared experience'

Published materials also carry a powerful message that this is not a unique experience. Sufficient numbers of people must have the same sorts of problem to warrant printing a leaflet or making a video. It helps break down the sense of isolation that can be so burdensome. They also ensure that there is consistency in what is being told. Modern multidisciplinary teams include a range of perspectives and levels of knowledge about illnesses and treatments and this can lead to confusion if the same questions receive differing answers from different members. Having common written materials reduces this risk. There is much to be gained in having an agreed team 'information pack' in the resource file for each disorder.

Blame and stigma

Increased understanding of the nature of the illness can go a long way to reducing the sense of guilt that is still so common in the families of young mentally ill adults. It is virtually inevitable that parents will search for an explanation of what caused the breakdown and all too often they come up with explanations based on how they brought up their child. Family life is never smooth and all of us can think of things we wish we had handled better and whose impact we probably exaggerate. Mothers in particular are prone to guilt and self-blame. They will be surrounded by friends and neighbours who believe that 'the parents are to blame' when young adults appear to go off the rails. Just because mental health professionals have examined closely and rejected family theories of causation of psychosis does not mean that this rejection is general. It is still important to be familiar with powerful folk-myths such as the 'schizophrenogenic mother' (Fromm-Reichmann 1948) and the 'double bind' (Bateson et al. 1956) in order to recognize them and refute them effectively.

Family support groups

Living with, and caring for, a young psychotic family member is a stressful and distressing experience. Modern community mental health services rely on families to be the main carers for patients. While the families generally welcome this, it is not without cost to them. Assessing the 'family burden' of caring for chronic illnesses has received extensive attention over the last 2–3 decades. With many disorders (e.g. Alzheimer's disease, arthritis, renal failure) there are tangible burdens that can be computed – time lost from paid work, time devoted to routine care (bathing, lifting, dressing etc.), opportunities lost (holidays, choice of accommodation) and so on. Many of these components of burden apply to the families of the mentally ill, but they are not the main issue.

Anticipatory care

The major part of the burden a severe mental illness imposes on a family comes from their emotional response to that illness. Time and energy is devoted to worrying about the patient and being alert to possible disasters ('anticipatory care'). Shame and fear of embarrassment contribute more to the isolation experienced by these families than time devoted to direct 'care'. There is a growing literature on this understanding of family burden in mental illness (Harvey et al. 2001) based on a stress-appraisal-coping paradigm (Szmukler et al. 1998). There are also several scales for assessing family burden with psychotic individuals (Pai and Kapur 1981; Schene et al. 1994; Szmukler et al. 1996).

Support

Undoubtedly there is a place for direct help to families of patients with psychotic illnesses as there is for those with physical illnesses. Home-help with cleaning and cooking can relieve some burden and the provision of transportation and respite undoubtedly improve the quality of life for families. However, just as the main burden derives from the appraisal of the illness, so effective relief is usually emotional and interpersonal. Breaking down the isolation and stigma felt by these families is what they report as most valuable. This is commonly achieved by open-ended support groups where they can meet others in the same situation.

Information

Often these groups involve an educational component (someone comes and gives a brief talk on some aspect of mental illness, new resources such as a job club or community facility are introduced to the group) but most of the time is spent exchanging experiences and supporting each other. New problem-solving skills can be acquired by learning how someone else deals with a similar situation with their child. Most importantly there is friendship and support and a realization that the tragedy of mental illness can afflict even the nicest and most generous of people. Nothing is more potent in the battle against guilt and self-imposed stigma than such peer support.

The importance of group support for families extends beyond simply how they feel. McFarlane (McFarlane *et al.* 1995) has shown that a group setting significantly increases the effect of behavioural family management in schizophrenia. The demoralization that families feel undercuts their problem-solving capacity. How they cope with the practical aspects of caring is highly responsive to support and encouragement.

Behavioural family management

The benefits of structured interventions to help families where there is high Expressed Emotion have been repeatedly confirmed (Mari and Streiner 1994; McCreadie *et al.* 1991; Pilling *et al.* 2002). This approach developed over 30 years ago (Brown *et al.* 1972) from attempts to understand why some schizophrenia patients on depot medication relapsed while most stayed well (Hirsch *et al.* 1973). Higher rates of relapse were linked to families with a particular interacting style which has come to be called 'high Expressed Emotion' (usually shortened to 'high EE'). This comprised explicit criticism, over-involvement and often overt hostility to the patient. Leff and his colleagues replicated the earlier findings and went on to show that an intervention could be developed that both reduced EE in the family and resulted in reduced relapse rates (Leff and Vaughn 1981; Willetts and Leff 1997). Although the research has been mainly conducted in established disorders there is little reason to question its value in first onset cases.

Behavioural Family Management in schizophrenia is now an accepted, evidence-based practice and one that is routinely taught in post-graduate nursing courses such as the Thorn course (Gournay and Birley 1998). It is a complex intervention that requires practice and skills training and for which there is extensive literature so it will not be further elaborated here. EIS teams need to ensure that these skills are available and routinely offered to families who need them. They usually build considerable expertise in BFM because, unlike other teams, so many of their patients still live with their families.

Relapse signature training

While there may be some controversy about the specificity of the prodromal syndrome there is none about the existence of 'early warning signs' of relapse in psychotic illnesses. Investigations have repeatedly confirmed that there are noticeable changes in mood, thinking, and behaviour which precede the emergence of frank psychosis (Birchwood *et al.* 1989, 2000; Jorgensen 1998). The Jorgensen and Birchwood (1989) studies even demonstrated good short-term prediction of relapse.

In bipolar disorder, manic relapse is often preceded by low level features of mania such as poor sleep and increasing energy which are still within the normal range but can be recognized as early warning signs (Perry *et al.* 1999). In schizophrenia the early warning signs are also often changes in mood – usually dysphoric (e.g. depression, rising tension, withdrawal, sleep disturbance) or a general sense of strangeness. Oversensitivity and suspiciousness are also common.

Management of early warning signs

Current understanding of schizophrenia and bipolar disorders draws heavily on the 'stress-vulnerability model' (Zubin and Spring 1977). From this it follows that the early warning signs are markers for rising stress in the individual. Stress, both in the form of life events (Hirsch *et al.* 1996) and intense family environments (Kuipers and Bebbington 1988), has been clearly shown to precipitate relapses in psychoses. Hogarty, a research social worker in the US, has built a whole treatment strategy based on the concept of 'affect dysregulation' (i.e. when the patient's mood becomes disorganized and out of control) which he believes is the mediator between increasing stress and relapse in schizophrenia (Hogarty *et al.* 1995).

The approaches to managing increasing stress include both psycho-social interventions and medication. Early attempts were made to replace maintenance medication in schizophrenia with so-called 'intermittent therapy' (where antipsychotics were introduced only when the patient showed early signs of relapsing). These were unsuccessful (Jolley *et al.* 1990). However, using low dose maintenance medication and increasing at first warning signs did seem relatively successful (Marder *et al.* 1984). It ensures that patients are exposed to less total quantities of drugs (Gaebel *et al.* 1993). The practice has not caught on because the gains seem outweighed by the uncertainties and clinical complexity.

Stress management using both behavioural strategies (e.g. avoidance, distraction) and cognitive behavioural treatments are receiving increasing attention. Patients often use such approaches without formal instruction. They learn to challenge emerging near-delusional ideas and to absent themselves from stressful situations (e.g. family meal-times). McCandless-Glimcher *et al.* (1986) consider these strategies to constitute self-taught cognitive behavioural therapy. More elaborate CBT exercises dealing with the meaning of symptoms to the patient have been found to be effective in established psychoses (Garety *et al.* 1994; Pilling *et al.* 2002) and there is currently interest in applying them to early warning signs.

Managing early warning signs

Recognizing early warning signs and using them to develop strategies to reduce relapse rates has been described in considerable detail.

Managing early warning signs

- Identification of relapse signature.
- Development of relapse drill.
- Rehearsal and monitoring.
- Clarification of relapse signature and drill.

Identification of relapse signature

If there is to be successful management of early warning signs they have to be recognized. While some signs are the same for most patients with specific disorders (e.g. poor sleep and increased energy before mania, tension, and withdrawal in schizophrenia) many individuals may have a specific 'relapse signature'. For some this may be very unusual and obvious, alerting family and staff. It is more important, however, for the *patient* to recognize impending relapse so that they can either introduce stress reduction strategies or seek help urgently.

Birchwood and his colleagues in Birmingham have evolved a highly acceptable strategy for working with individual patients to identify their relapse signature and develop a response (Birchwood *et al.* 2000). There are two main steps to the process:

1. Time line exercise
2. Card sort exercise

Time line exercise

The patient is encouraged to review with their key worker the months before referral to the mental health services and to describe their experiences and feelings. While doing this they try and identify what was going on at the time – both in their own lives and in general. By 'pegging' these experiences to current affairs and significant events the patient is able to form an understanding of the sequence of internal experiences and a sense of the time scale of the process.

Card sort exercise

Based on clinical experience and published literature 55 features commonly cited as occurring before relapse are printed in large font, each on an individual laminated card. These are examined with the patient who can say whether or not they have had that particular experience. Those that are identified as relevant are spread out on a table and arranged in various ways. They are first arranged in order of onset so that they reflect the time sequence. Some may be then recognized as clustering together and are put in groups. Patients can propose other warning signs that are not included in the set and these are written on similar cards. Working with the cards is not just a one-off exercise – the therapist and patient discuss them at length, try to understand them, link them to stressors, try and locate the threshold where insight is lost etc. They are used then to construct a relapse drill. The whole process can take up to six sessions.

Early warning signs of psychotic relapse – card sort exercise

Thinking/perception	Feelings	Behaviours
◆ Thoughts are racing	◆ Feeling helpless or useless	◆ Difficulty sleeping
◆ Senses seem sharper	◆ Feeling afraid of going crazy	◆ Speech comes out jumbled filled with odd words
◆ Thinking you have special powers	◆ Feeling sad or low	◆ Talking or smiling to yourself
◆ Thinking that you can read other people's minds	◆ Feeling anxious and restless	◆ Acting suspiciously as if being watched
◆ Thinking that other people can read your mind	◆ Feeling increasingly religious	◆ Behaving oddly for no reason
◆ Receiving personal messages from the TV or radio	◆ Feeling like you are being watched	◆ Spending time alone
◆ Having difficulty making decisions	◆ Feeling isolated	◆ Neglecting your appearance
◆ Experiencing strange sensations	◆ Feeling tired or lacking energy	◆ Acting like you are somebody else
◆ Preoccupied about 1 or 2 things	◆ Feeling confused or puzzled	◆ Not seeing people
◆ Thinking you might be somebody else	◆ Feeling forgetful or far away	◆ Not eating

Early warning signs of psychotic relapse – card sort exercise *(continued)*

Thinking/perception	Feelings	Behaviours
◆ Seeing visions or things others cannot see	◆ Feeling in another world	◆ Not leaving the house
◆ Thinking people are talking about you	◆ Feeling strong and powerful	◆ Behaving like a child
◆ Thinking people are against you	◆ Feeling unable to cope with everyday tasks	◆ Refusing to do simple requests
◆ Having more nightmares	◆ Feeling like you are just being punished	◆ Drinking more
◆ Having difficulty concentrating	◆ Feeling like you cannot trust other people	◆ Smoking more ◆ Movements are slow
◆ Thinking bizarre things	◆ Feeling irritable	◆ Unable to sit down for long
◆ Thinking your thoughts are controlled	◆ Feeling like you do not need sleep	◆ Behaving aggressively
◆ Hearing voices	◆ Feeling guilty	
◆ Thinking that a part of you has changed shape		

Reproduced from "Schizophrenia: early warning signs" (Birchwood et al. 2000)

Developing a relapse drill

The relapse drill is a three-stage action plan which is developed from the relapse signature.

1. *Staging of warning signs:*
   - *Pathways to support* – details of how to contact services both within and outside office hours.
   - *Service interventions* – increased contact, anxiety/stress management, agreed temporary increase in medications, respite care or home treatment.
   - *Personal coping strategies* – coping strategies which the patient has discovered for themselves or is taught.
2. *Rehearsal and monitoring.*
3. *Clarification of signature and drill.*

Staging

In 'staging' the early warning signs identified in the card sort and time line exercise are classified into early, middle, and late based on the previous relapse. Each group is then associated with specific strategies and interventions that can protect the patient from progressing further down the pathway to psychosis. The early signs (dysphoric and anxiety-related features) are most often the non-specific – i.e. they may simply be part and parcel of normal life and recede. With these the interventions tend to be life-style alterations – avoiding stress, distraction etc. As the warning signs progress to the later ones, more likely to predict relapse, specific, trained coping strategies are used (such as CBT procedures to challenge over-valued ideas). With more specific early warning signs (e.g. disturbed sleep and withdrawal, brief but frankly psychotic symptoms) stepping up contact frequency with the team and increasing antipsychotic medication is indicated.

This staging process (like everything in the relapse-drill planning) is a collaborative venture between caseworker and patient and the educational benefits for both parties cannot be overstated. Both get to understand the details of the patient's illness in real depth. Careful staging of response is probably a counsel of perfection. Most teams, in practice, move quite quickly to using an increase in monitoring and then medication.

Rehearsal and monitoring

When things are going wrong is not the best time try new approaches. The relapse drill needs to be practised so that the patient and family feel confident for when they might really need it. Both patient and family should receive their own copies of the relapse prevention form and various scenarios can be rehearsed and played out with the case manager. Such role-plays help 'lighten up' the relationship and are generally enjoyed by all involved. They can also spot possible problems that might otherwise prevent the intervention being effective.

Clarifying and reviewing the signature and drill

Simply constructing and providing a document is not enough in itself. The process is dynamic and needs regular review and updating. If not it will be forgotten. New and more successful coping strategies are likely to be developed as the patient and family gain greater confidence and understanding of the illness, and as the therapeutic relationship strengthens. Each time the relapse drill is activated (at whatever level) then it should be reviewed and used as a learning experience to improve it.

Problems with relapse drills

Birchwood (2000) identifies some common problems with constructing a relapse strategy.

Lack of insight

The most obvious is when insight into the process is absent or lost very early and the patient does not recognize that the changes have any pathological meaning. Insight is a tricky concept – it is not a simple on–off state. It may be partial and lack of insight can even be necessary for preserving self-esteem. It is common for young people to insist that their 'breakdown' was entirely the consequence of drugs, or that it was a 'spiritual journey'. This denial may be both impenetrable and beneficial in many ways. The challenge is still to identify features of the process of breakdown and propose interventions without using them to contradict the patient's (and sometimes family's) construction of events. It serves to remind us that our task is to work with the patient to reduce the disruption of psychosis – not to prove their delusions wrong.

Losing insight

Some patients develop insight but lose it very rapidly at the start of a breakdown. This is common with bipolar disorder where the 'window of opportunity' is often very narrow between the emergence of the first warning signs and the established denial typical of elation. McGorry and McConville (1999) describe patients who, despite developing 'past insight', lose 'present insight'. These patients can construct their relapse plan when they look back on what happened but as soon as they start to get ill again it all evaporates. Birchwood recommends increased efforts to involve the family in this group and also to make routine prospective monitoring of early warning signs an explicit part of the care package.

Sealing over

McGlashan (McGlashan *et al.* 1975) has tried to define what he calls 'recovery style'. By this he means how individuals deal with the memory of a traumatic episode such as a psychosis. It has become popular to encourage individuals with all sorts of difficult experiences (e.g. after car crashes, or with a terminal diagnosis) to confront and accept the implications and 'work-through' the experience to obtain resolution. This approach of openness and emotional honesty fits the tenor of our times although, in many instances, the evidence is against it.

Possible health value of 'sealing over'

Careful studies of victims of life-threatening trauma (Bisson *et al.* 2000; Hobbs *et al.* 1996; Mayou *et al.* 2000; Raphael and Meldrum 1995) have confirmed the folk wisdom which advises confronting the situation but denying the anxiety ('*get back on the horse as soon as possible*'). Figure 5.3 from a study of traffic accidents (Mayou *et al.* 2000) shows that the recovery of highly traumatized traffic accident victims was *delayed* by counselling. Those left alone were over it by four months. These more recent findings have more implications for crisis resolution teams (Chapter 6), but cannot be ignored in EIS teams.

Working with psychosis, an informed collaborative relationship between patient and care staff is the only real hope of remaining well. Not confronting and talking through the experience of the illness poses real problems so, despite this contrary evidence, there is little scope for avoiding the issues.

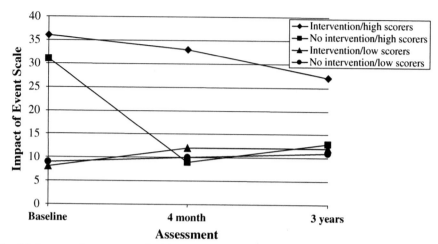

Fig. 5.3 Impact of event scores for high and low scores in intervention and no-intervention group at baseline assessment, 4-month and 3-year follow-ups (Mayer *et al.* 2000)

Acknowledging the illness without excessive preoccupation

A persisting paradox is that real quality of life for our patients often depends on being able to 'forget about' their illnesses and get on with normal life; yet if they neglect their illness management then they have simply no chance of achieving this. Dealing with patients who 'seal over' encapsulates this dilemma. Examination of early warning signs with this group may, indeed, be experienced as confrontational, be counter-productive and generate increased anxiety. The answer may lie in timing – waiting until the therapeutic relationship is stronger, and the fear of relapse less, before embarking on a relapse plan. Sometimes it simply cannot be done.

Lack of syndrome stability

Interest in relapse signatures has lead many to believe that individual relapse signatures are the norm and can always be identified. This is not the case. Especially when working in EIS teams (where there may be only one or two previous breakdowns to examine) it is often difficult to identify individual patterns with any certainty. Individuals may also experience very different features before successive breakdowns. This should not surprise us – people learn and change. Their increased understanding and experience of the illness affects their response, their personal circumstances change and there are other external influences. Alcohol and drug use are potent distortions of the signature. Similarly the response to a previous episode (McGorry 1994) is bound to affect the build up to a subsequent one (whether it is increased apprehension, denial, or dismay).

Conclusions

Relapse signature training has been dealt with at great length here because it is one of the activities that EIS teams have developed so successfully. The approach is equally relevant, however, to all teams – perhaps even more relevant to assertive outreach teams for patients with long established illnesses and frequent relapses. The incorporation of the technique should be actively considered by these other teams.

There has been a tendency to exaggerate the potential of this approach and some of the difficulties have been outlined above. However this is not to deny the real promise it offers. Not only is it likely that it can reduce relapse rates but earlier intervention should ameliorate those relapses that do occur. More importantly it embodies a whole-person, collaborative approach in a most direct and obvious manner for patients, families and staff. It is less sophisticated and daunting than many of the other psycho-social interventions and one that should take a central place in the team's repertoire.

'Recovery' programmes

Coming to terms with their diagnosis is a challenge all young adults face after the first psychotic breakdown. EIS teams have pioneered an emphasis on what are often called 'recovery' programmes. These are structured approaches to helping the individual acknowledge the reality of their illness while they focus on their recovery. The approach emphasizes psychological understanding of the experience. Usually a clinical psychologist takes referrals from the case manager. Recovery work is usually modular.

Components of recovery work

- Problem lists.
- Recovery proper (CBT approach).
- Recovery group.

All patients are offered the basic 4–5 sessions working on problem lists and understanding their illness. Most take up this offer. All are also offered the more long term and extensive CBT programme (a flexible 20 sessions over 3 years) but only about a third take this up. A slow-open recovery group is offered to both those who engage with the CBT and also to those who only work on the problem lists. The group is fairly informal and is a mix of psychoeducation, coping, and recovery.

Cognitive behaviour therapy and problem solving therapies

There is a growing literature on the use of cognitive behaviour therapy and a variety of short-term psychological therapies aimed at improving interpersonal problem solving for use with psychotic patients. CBT for persistent delusions and distressing hallucinations is probably the best known of these interventions (Chadwick and Birchwood 1994;

Jackson *et al.* 1998; Kingdon and Turkington 1994; Pilling *et al.* 2002). It must not be forgotten, however, that EIS teams are often dealing with very young people who face stressful developmental issues which are not all part of the illness. This is a time in life when establishing identity, moving further away from parents and perhaps settling with a partner face everyone. Targeted psychotherapies such as Cognitive Analytic Therapy (CAT) (Ryle and Kerr 2002), Interpersonal Therapy (Weissman and Markowitz 1994) or even psychosis-specific psychotherapies such as personal therapy (Hogarty *et al.* 1997) can all contribute.

All of these therapies require training to acquire the necessary skills and courses exist to provide this training for CMHT staff (Gournay and Birley 1998). Because of their style and their relatively high resourcing EIS teams have generally been more vigorous in getting such training and applying it within their service. However they are just as relevant to other teams dealing with psychotic patients. The individual techniques will not be outlined in detail here – those wishing to know more can enquire locally about training opportunities.

Vikram, a 20-year-old man of Indian origin, has a recent onset but treatment-resistant psychosis with persistent command hallucinations and disabling social anxiety despite Clozapine treatment. He lives in an emotional family with an overprotective mother and a domineering father, who attributes Vikram's symptoms to 'laziness'. The family has been reluctant to be involved in systematic behavioural intervention. A CBT programme was initiated, which involved learning cognitive techniques to manage his hallucinatory experiences, and a behavioural programme of daily travel outside the home with a support worker from the team. Over 6 months, Vikram mastered cognitive remediation strategies for dealing with his hallucinations and was able to spend time out of home on his own. After a further six-months attendance at a youth project where he received computer training, he found employment with a local shop. He continues to hold a part-time job despite continuing hallucinations and the family environment has settled markedly.

Vocational rehabilitation

Much of the motivation behind establishing EIS teams was that it is in the early stages of psychosis that patients lose most in terms of their social functioning. Patients who drop out of work or education during their first breakdown have very low rates of re-entry to either the job market or college. The longer they remain out of the mainstream (even when active symptoms have remitted) the less likely they are to make up lost ground. As a consequence most EIS teams include a vocational counsellor or, at the very least, identify a team member with special responsibility for vocational support and placement.

Individual placement service

The model of vocational service that is currently most favoured is that of seeking an early placement for the patient in a fairly undemanding ('entry level') job and supporting both the patient and the employer in it. This *'place and train'* approach is in contrast to previous '*train and place*' models. These latter involved extensive job training within the mental health services to equip patients with the skills to acquire and retain jobs. The place and train approach is most clearly articulated in the IPS (Individual Placement Service) approach to supported employment (Becker and Drake 1993). There are now two large scale trials which have demonstrated the superiority of this approach in the US over conventional vocational rehabilitation (Drake *et al.* 1999; Lehman 1995; Lehman *et al.* 2002). Although it remains to be shown that this approach is successful outside the US or when unemployment levels are high, its current place as the model of choice is not in dispute.

EIS teams aim for rapid job search and keep the prospect of return to education or work high on the clinical agenda. Consequently (see above) they are less concerned to maximize welfare benefits, particularly where these can lock the patient into long-term dependency and remove the incentive to get work (Turton 2001). There is no doubt that the main incentive to work for young patients is money. Staff may stress gains in self-esteem, a structured day, company etc., but patients rarely rate these. They want money to buy decent clothes and get out and about like their peers. Once they are without a job for any length of time, and give up on this desire for the same quality of life as those around them, then it can be a long road back.

Responsibility for inpatient care

EIS teams aim to reduce hospitalization to a minimum. In this they are no different from other CMHTs but admission can be particularly traumatic for young people. Admission to an acute psychiatric ward is never easy. The very success of community mental health care has meant that wards now contain only the most severely ill patients. Many will be there involuntarily. They are often quite scary places, full of strangers, many of whom are angry and hostile.

Coping with this stressful environment for any patient draws on both the support the staff can offer but also the individual patient's own resilience and sense of identity. Young people who are still struggling to develop a sense of 'who they are' may find the ward particularly unsettling. This has always been a problem for adolescents admitted to adult wards. The PIG guidance is singularly unhelpful in this context stating blithely that if hospitalization is needed: 'Separate age, gender and culture appropriate accommodation should be provided.'

Where to admit severely ill young patients

In reality severely ill young patients will be admitted to whichever ward can cope with them. A high proportion of first episode patients continue to be admitted to hospital even in the best services. In the LEO service's first two years of operation over 90% of patients had at least one admission – often at first presentation. Their goal is to reduce this to the Melbourne service's level of about 55%. However, admission remains, and will remain, a significant feature of EIS.

Many will be admitted against their will and to Psychiatric Intensive Care Units. Currently adolescent services have very restricted abilities to admit highly disturbed young psychotic patients. The pros and cons of admitting to a distant adolescent unit (often out of district) or to a less appropriate adult unit (but which is nearby, where they can retain contact with family members and the care team) has to be weighed carefully. Local circumstances will play a major role – in rural areas such as the Highlands of Scotland the nearest adolescent unit may be a hundred miles away whereas in London travelling may not be a major issue. Similarly if the local adult unit is well run and can offer an individual room and individual nursing to the young patient, or if there is a well functioning women only ward available for an adolescent girl, this will influence the decision. This is not an area for dogmatism. Clinical judgement must be applied on a case-by-case basis.

Respite units

Several services have developed small admission facilities which are domestic in atmosphere, have limited staffing and are established away from the hospital. These are often converted houses or perhaps located in a resource centre. Usually they admit up to 6–8 patients (some are even smaller) for periods of weeks when they are too unwell to remain at home (or need some targeted rehabilitation). In many ways they reflect the approach of the better Italian services (Chapter 8).

Types of respite units

The level of staffing and degree of disturbance tolerated in respite units both vary considerably. Some are registered as part of the hospital so that they can accommodate involuntary patients while others are run by housing associations with staff provided by the health services. There is no agreed optimal model and they probably differ as much from each other as they do from traditional inpatient units. Those which take patients for short periods overlap in character with crisis houses (Sledge et al. 1995) and those which take patients for longer, including involuntary patients, are more like hospital hostels (Brook 1973) both of which have extensive literatures.

These less-institutional settings are generally much more acceptable to younger patients. Those who work in them report that residents respond to the more personal atmosphere and exhibit significantly less disturbed behaviour. It is, of course, difficult to know how much confidence to attach to this observation. Those patients likely to be the most disturbed are probably directed away from the respite unit to the admission ward. However a significant reduction in disturbed behaviour and the rate of compulsion has been noted in two newly built non-selective units in East London which offered improved facilities and privacy.

The process of admission to these respite facilities seems less drastic in some way. Patients will often be admitted for a few days or a week or so if tension at home is raised or they need increased support. As a consequence it is not unusual for residents to carry on going to college or working from them.

Drug and alcohol use

There are tricky problems with alcohol and substance abuse in this group. It is hard to abide by simple rules and regulations – a delicate balance has to be struck between tolerance to promote engagement and rigor for ensuring safety for all involved and, indeed, respect for the law of the land. Most units take a very serious view of any drug dealing on the premises and will consider it as a strong indication for early discharge. However some level of drug use and alcohol consumption is almost inevitable with this patient group. Where intoxication leads to profound difficulties with treatment or risk to other patients then tough clinical decisions may be needed about more secure settings.

Relationships with inpatient services and other teams

Responsibility for inpatient care

Discontinuity of care is generally to be avoided with severely ill individuals. Care will have to transfer between teams when it is simply not possible for the current team to provide the necessary levels of skill or intensity. Whether care should transfer wholly when patients are admitted differs internationally. In many European countries this is the preferred model and strong arguments are advanced for it (citing concentration of appropriate skills and focusing of responsibility). In the UK there has been a strong preference for the CMHT retaining responsibility for inpatient care (Chapter 3). This may not be the case where the Home Treatment team is the gateway to inpatient care and manages the admission (Department of Health 2002).

There is no certainty about the right approach here – and certainly no research evidence to base it upon. Current UK policy is to encourage the management of admissions by the Home Treatment Team but in practice there is a kaleidoscope of arrangements. EIS teams which have their own respite units tend to retain full responsibility and inreach throughout those admissions. Some teams also have their own admission ward beds and some use beds 'belonging' to routine CMHTs. LEO has its own large admission unit, which is central to its identity and functioning. How the EIS relates to inpatient care will depend on the service structure it adopts and, in particular, how thinly spread it is (Singh *et al.* 2002).

Relationships with other teams in the local service

The same uncertainty about how the EIS team relates to inpatient care is likely to be true for how it relates to the other components of the local services. It would be misleading to suggest that there is any consensus on the fine details of how EIS teams relate to teams around them. It is unsafe to make such assumptions. Local arrangements need to be hammered out with all the relevant stakeholders (CMHTs, wards, GPs etc), to be crystal clear, to be *mutually* agreed and to be written down. Given the current rapid developments with EIS teams these arrangements should be subject to regular revision by all those involved and checked out with other EIS teams to identify emerging good practice.

Relationships with other teams should be

- Crystal clear.
- Locally agreed.
- Mutually agreed.
- Written down.
- Regularly reviewed.

Conclusions

Of all the new specialized CMHTs, Early Intervention Teams are the most difficult to describe. This is because they are the most varied and often lead by strikingly charismatic leaders who rarely dwell on uncertainties in practice. As a result the differences between them can be vast. These are not just minor differences about how often the team meets or what documentation they use. They are fundamental differences about who the team is for, the extent of its remit, the interventions offered and, indeed, their whole ideology and atmosphere. The current tendency to skate over these differences and imply that there is an accepted consistent model of the EIS team is misleading and unhelpful.

For ease of understanding three major components have been presented as separate teams (which they may, or may not, be):

- Continuing care (AO team).
- Outreach and detection team.
- Prodromal treatment team.

This last is a controversial, experimental approach to treating high-risk individuals before they have fully developed the disorder. In many ways this apparent confusion is very healthy and should be welcomed. It will allow the development and identification over time of the really effective and efficient structures.

EIS teams encapsulate a new optimism within community mental health. Their motivation really is to improve the quality of life of young people at this most distressing and vulnerable period of their illness. They have, thankfully, not been established to save money by reducing hospital care, nor to reduce risk to the population by keeping 'dangerous' patients engaged. They exist to provide a broad, humane approach to both patients and families so that they can survive the awful experience of a first psychotic episode. Time will tell whether a separate service really is needed to achieve this. Inevitably, however, the high standards they set should begin to be the benchmarks for all services for psychotic individuals, which can only be to the good.

CHAPTER 6

Crisis resolution and home treatment teams

Crisis intervention theory and the history of crisis teams

Crisis is a concept applied widely in human discourse. It implies that a system under stress has reached the limits of its flexibility, and if the stress continues then either it will break down or have to change radically. It is regularly applied in economic and political contexts where crises are often seen as the catalysts of major (often revolution-ary) change. Crisis is a dynamic concept and not necessarily a negative one – the Chinese Ideogram for Crisis is famously made up of the symbols for both 'threat' and 'opportunity'. In the emotional lives of individuals it has this connotation of a cross-roads – a phase in personal development which is dramatic in intensity and whose out-come is uncertain.

The Chinese Ideogram for 'Crisis'

"Whenever there is danger, there are opportunities."

There is a sense that after a crisis things cannot simply be the same again. In a suc-cessful resolution the individual may be changed in some significant way ('sadder but wiser', 'more mature'). Crises may be survived, though at a cost, such as in bereavement where we return to normal functioning but often are never fully the same again. Lastly crises can be so overwhelming that individuals simply do not recover.

Life events and crises

We are subject to stresses throughout our lives. The enormous physical and hormonal upheavals of adolescence and pregnancy, or disability in later life, are examples of 'developmental' crises. Eric Erikson (Erikson 1959) emphasized these developmental challenges and saw mastery of them as the key to personal well-being and growth.

'Accidental' crises can vary from the spectacular (e.g. floods and earthquakes) to the domestic (e.g. redundancy, moving house). Often referred to as 'life events', they have long been known to affect mental health and to precipitate breakdowns – even ranked according to their 'stressfulness' (Holmes and Rahe 1967; Paykel 1997) – and regularly found to precede relapses in major mental illnesses (Bebbington *et al.* 1993; Kendler *et al.* 1995; Paykel 1978). Paradoxically so-called 'positive events' (such as promotion or marriage) are also stressful. Events which involve loss ('exit-events') have, unsurprisingly, been shown to be particularly potent in precipitating depression.

Crisis intervention theory

In 1942, Coconut Grove (a night-club in the US town of Boston) burnt down with the loss of 491 young lives. A number of psychiatrists worked with the bereaved and from this experience Lindemann (Lindemann 1944) developed a theory of crisis intervention. Lindemann was struck by how rapidly he gained emotional access to conflict and distress in the families of victims, and how comparatively easy it was to promote change and resolution. He concluded that most of the work expended in, the then current, psychoanalytical therapy was absorbed in overcoming fixed, psychological defence mechanisms to get to the underlying conflicts. In crisis patients these defence mechanisms had been breached and so the therapist was able to work directly with the core problems.

Transitional states

Lindemann believed that crises arose when habitual psychological defence mechanisms were overwhelmed – a crisis was when the usual responses did not work, even when at full stretch. New responses had to be developed quickly or collapse was imminent. Lindemann, and subsequently Caplan (Caplan 1961), became convinced that crises offered unique opportunities for psychological growth and effective intervention. Their 'Crisis Theory' had a series of 'transitional states' of which Lindemann emphasized early '*recoil*' and Caplan '*emotional homeostasis*' and '*hazards*'. Influenced by Erikson's up-beat approach to developmental crises they advanced crisis intervention not only as an effective treatment of mental health problems but as a powerful force for personal growth and primary prevention of psychiatric disorders (Fig. 6.1).

Reappraisal of crisis theory

Much of this initial enthusiasm for crisis theory has waned. Evidence for primary prevention (i.e. preventing the development of a disorder altogether) did not materialize. Even more disappointing (as addressed in Chapter 5), there has been evidence that crisis work can sometimes hamper the normal healing process and make things worse (Bisson *et al.* 2000; Hobbs *et al.* 1996; Mayou *et al.* 2000; Wessely *et al.* 1998). Consequently recent crisis writings have focused on reducing the impact of crises on the individual rather than seeking to promote personal development.

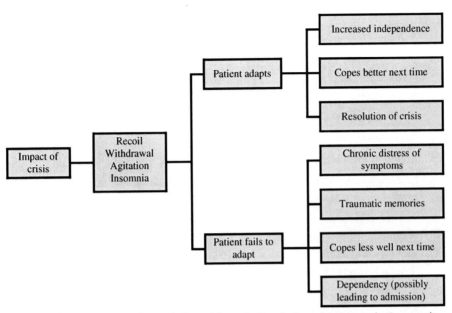

Fig. 6.1 Theoretical stages of crisis (Adapted from H. Katschnig and J. Cooper in Community Psychiatry (Katschnig and Cooper 1991))

Post traumatic stress disorder (PTSD)

Post Traumatic Stress Disorder (PTSD) is the term that is currently applied to a persisting emotional reaction to severe stress (American Psychiatric Association 1994) (World Health Organization 1992). Although most individuals do get over awful experiences there is a proportion who continue to be over-aroused and preoccupied with them. Their descriptions of persisting nightmares, vivid intrusive memories of the event, poor concentration, and heightened emotionality (in particular a tendency to 'startle' reactions) is remarkably consistent. The diagnosis is made when the condition lasts more than a month and the diagnostic features are:

DSM-IV criteria for PTSD (American Psychiatric Association 1994)

A:

1. Experienced, witnessed or confronted with an event, or events, that involved actual or threatened death or serious injury, or a threat to the physical integrity of self or others.

2. The person's response involved intense fear, helplessness, or horror.

DSM-IV criteria for PTSD (American Psychiatric Association 1994) *(continued)*

B: The traumatic event is persistently re-experienced in one (or more) of the following ways:

1. Recurrent and intrusive distressing recollections of the event, including images, thoughts, or perceptions.

2. Recurrent distressing dreams of the event.

3. Acting or feeling as if the traumatic event were recurring.

4. Intense psychological distress at exposure to internal or external cues that symbolize or resemble an aspect of the traumatic event.

5. Physiological reactivity at exposure to internal or external cues.

C: Persistent avoidance of stimuli associated with the trauma and numbing of general responsiveness (not present before), as indicated by three or more of the following:

1. Efforts to avoid thoughts, feelings, or conversations associated with the trauma.

2. Efforts to avoid places, or people that arouse recollections of the trauma.

3. Inability to recall an important aspect of the trauma.

4. Markedly diminished interest or participation in significant activities.

5. Feeling of detachment or estrangement from others.

6. Restricted range of affect.

7. Sense of foreshortened future.

D: Persistent symptoms of increased arousal as indicated by two (or more) of following:

1. Difficulty falling asleep.

2. Irritability or outbursts of anger.

3. Difficulty concentrating.

4. Hypervigilance.

5. Exaggerated startle response.

Treatment of straightforward 'acute' PTSD was initially restricted to counselling but in more severe cases both cognitive behavioural therapy and psychodynamic psychotherapy have been shown to be useful (Van Etten and Taylor 1998). Pharmacological treatments (mainly antidepressants and short term benzodiazepines (Davidson 1997)) have also been shown to work as have short courses of 'Eye Movement desensitization and Reprocessing' (EMDR) (Shapiro and Maxfield 2002).

Controversies and uncertainties around PTSD

This 'simple' PTSD outlined above is an easily recognizable disorder that has had many names over the decades (e.g. delayed shock, acute stress disorder, battle fatigue). However the diagnosis and concept have been muddied by use with the long-term behavioural and personality difficulties initially described in Vietnam veterans. It has become even more diffuse with the proposal of complex PTSD (Herman 1992) as an explanation of persisting and entrenched personality difficulties, and social and psychological impairment. Summerfield has even questioned the concept altogether, insisting that it medicalizes natural responses to tragedies deflecting attention from effective social responses (Summerfield 1999, 2001).

Relevance of PTSD to modern crisis resolution teams

Although PTSD and psychological debriefing are often alluded to in literature, about crisis services neither are central to current thinking on crisis resolution teams. Both PTSD management and psychological debriefing are generally the remit of specialists. Most emergency services (e.g. firefighters, police) have their own debriefing arrangements. Forensic psychiatry's focus on victimology has encompassed PTSD and its treatment.

Probably the two major contributions of PTSD to crisis teams are the recognition of over-arousal and the need to deal with predisposing and risk factors simultaneously with the current situation. Over-arousal is common in the early phase of any rapid, stressful change (e.g. the patients' and families' experience of a psychotic relapse). Time and reassurance are both essential components in any treatment approach. Similarly background issues may be crucial in making an individual vulnerable to a breakdown in a crisis when otherwise they would have coped. The crisis may simply be 'the straw that broke the camel's back' and assessments must avoid an oversimplified and narrow causality.

Ronald was a 43-year-old electrician admitted to an orthopaedic ward after a train crash in which over 30 people had been killed just before Christmas. He sustained multiple fractures to his legs plus several broken ribs and overall, though not at risk of dying, he was in considerable pain.

He was one of several victims of the crash on the ward and became increasingly distressed over the weeks of his long admission. At interview he displayed all the features of PTSD, with terrifying flashbacks of regaining consciousness in the carriage alongside a young woman who died slowly from bleeding before they could be freed. She repeatedly cried out for her two children. In trying to deal with the enormous distress he was experiencing (and his anger and shame at not being able to control it) the psychologist took a broad history, not just focusing on the disaster. The issue of Ronald's son who was adopted away at birth many years ago surfaced again and again in their sessions. Eventually, as things seemed to be deteriorating rather than improving, she encouraged him to talk more about these earlier events ("so that I can get a better understanding of who you are").

His response was dramatic. He poured out the misery that he had sealed up for years about this adoption, which he had not really wanted, and which was then compounded by their failure to have any children when they did marry. The dying woman's longing for her children broke through his long established defences. What blocked him dealing with the horror of his experience was some vague (and to him, shocking and distasteful) feeling that 'at least she had had children'. Ventilating and recognising these thoughts allowed him to then get on with dealing with his PTSD.

Crisis resolution and home treatment teams

This reappraisal of crisis theory has brought greater realism about the benefits and limitations of crisis intervention. It has not been abandoned, far from it, we have retained an understanding of the role of support during times of crisis. Individuals with strong support networks (especially supportive families) cope much better with all sorts of crises (even survival in concentration camps was much higher in those in families or who were members of a tight-knit group). The period of emotional disequilibrium in a crisis is a dangerous and distressing one. Modern crisis services aim to shorten and contain it with support and, if indicated, specific treatments.

However neither classical crisis theory nor PTSD are the main drivers for the establishment of Crisis Resolution and Home Treatment (CR/HT) teams. Two powerful forces are currently responsible for their prominence.

Users' and carers' voices

Organizations representing patients and their families repeatedly emphasize the need for rapid access at times of distress. 'Who can we get hold of when things are falling apart?' is the common cry, usually expressed as 'who will be there in the middle of the night?'. The failure of many services to provide prompt routine access to patients and their families explains the strength of this demand. All too many services operate waiting lists for routine appointments and many offer no facility for a rapid, urgent assessment other than a visit to A&E or a brief domicilliary visit by the consultant.

Comparisons with medical emergency services

This emphasis on a rapid response is strengthened by comparisons with emergency services in general medicine – e.g. cardiac resuscitation by paramedics in specially equipped ambulances which arrive within minutes. The idea of the 'life threatening emergency' transfers easily across from cardiology to psychiatry although, in truth, there is no mental health equivalent of a heart attack. This equivalence of services encapsulates the legitimate desire to reduce discrimination between mental and physical healthcare.

Poor local provision

Patchy and variable services legitimize the consumerist demands of patients and families for crisis services. If an urgent need is neglected it will eventually become an emergency. Health care provision has increasingly embraced the merits of consumerism, and probably rightly so. Despite the evidence of low use of crisis services (especially at night) even when they are provided, the vivid experience of *no* help being offered at times of great distress carries the argument. Some form of immediate access needs to be provided and that provision must not be grudging. The availability of some crisis provision also acts as a reassurance such that it is not needed. Knowing that help is at hand can make the anxiety manageable.

Reduction in bed use

Crisis resolution and home treatment (CR/HT) teams are also promoted to reduce reliance on inpatient care. The last 50 years has seen a steady reduction in the use of inpatient care in mental health, particularly long-term inpatient care. This is a development to be welcomed – most patients and their families express a clear wish to stay in their own homes if adequate help can be provided. The disruption to family life of admission is an added burden to an individual already struggling with a mental illness. The loss of family support can be keenly felt at such a vulnerable time. As well as the benefits to the patient of being able to remain at home, the service benefits by being able to devote more of its limited resources to community care. Inpatient care is still prohibitively expensive and absorbs a disproportionate fraction of mental health care spend.

Equivocal evidence of bed reduction

CR/HT teams have been advocated for their ability to reduce hospital admissions (Smyth and Hoult 2000). It is undoubtedly the case that there have been several high profile examples of bed usage rapidly reducing with the introduction of a crisis resolution or home treatment service (Hoult *et al.* 1984; Dean *et al.* 1993; Stefansson and Cullberg 1986). However there are good reasons to be cautious in interpreting these results (Burns 2000*a*; Coid 1994). In several instances the crisis service was introduced into a 'failing' system as part of a new broom. It may be difficult to distinguish the benefits of the home treatment approach from the quality and commitment of the new staff (particularly highly motivated senior doctors and nurses) (Coid 1994). It is still far from clear that the dramatic reductions in bed use reported in some of these high profile studies will be replicated when they are introduced into otherwise well-functioning services.

Time will tell if routine crisis services do, or do not, significantly alter inpatient occupancy. For the individual patient, however, bed reduction is not the issue. For them what matters is whether they can get rapid and effective help.

Who are CR/HT teams for?

The Policy Implementation Guide (Department of Health 2001) is explicit about the target population for CR/HT teams:

> Commonly adults (16 to 65 years old) with severe mental illness (schizophrenia, manic depressive disorders, severe depressive disorder) with an acute psychiatric crisis of such severity that, without the involvement of the CR/HT team hospitalization would be necessary.

Not only is the Implementation guide explicit about who it is for, it is equally forth-right about who should *not* be treated by it:

The service is not usually appropriate for individuals with:

- Mild anxiety disorders.
- Primary diagnosis of alcohol or other substance abuse.
- Brain damage or other organic disorders including dementia.
- Learning disabilities.
- Exclusive diagnosis of personality disorder.
- Recent history of self harm but not suffering from a psychotic or serious depressive illness.
- Crisis related solely to relationship issues.

Anyone working in an acute mental health service will know that this is a counsel of perfection. In reality you will not know till you have seen the patient whether this is a serious disorder or not. Many of the crises which do not meet these very stringent criteria (e.g. self-harm patients or those with situational anxiety states) will often present the opportunity for extremely effective brief counselling (perhaps requiring just 2–3 sessions) that are rewarding to the patient and the staff alike. It is impractical (and usually fruitless) to refer them on, and inhumane to refuse a follow-up or two.

Not 'widening the net'

However this definition of the target population gives an unequivocal steer to the team. It confirms that this is *not about widening the net* but offering a crisis service to the same group of patients who currently would be dealt with on enhanced CPA in traditional CMHTs (i.e. severe or enduring mental illness). Similarly the phrase '...*without the involvement of the CR/HT team, hospitalization would be necessary*' indicates the level of severity of disorder.

Current CR/HT teams have learnt from early crisis services (Cooper 1979) that without explicit targeting they will be overwhelmed by inappropriate referrals – predominantly relationship and alcohol issues. Where CR/HT teams take referrals from beyond secondary care mental health teams, inappropriate ones are inevitable. The South Islington team in London (a well-established team able to give a comprehensive account of its practice) still sees a significant proportion of intoxicated patients in A&E. Educating referrers can go so far, but a willingness to assess briefly and give an opinion (even, or especially, if it is 'no involvement with mental health services indicated') remains an essential component of the good CR/HT team's function.

Use of triage

Some CR/HT teams share a 'triage' function with an open access telephone crisis helpline provided in the district. As most of the referrals will come by telephone there is some merit in structuring the referral information. This allows less experienced staff to man the lines, but also provides increasing information about how the local crisis services are being used. Such information is the basis for reviewing and refining service provision over time. Figure 6.2 is an example of such an initial contact sheet used by a telephone crisis line. As remarked in Chapter 2, care needs to be exercised with such structured data collection as callers generally dislike being 'forced' to give structured information when what they want to do is tell their story.

How long is a crisis?

When does crisis care merge into routine care in severe mental illness? Most severe mental illnesses are relapsing-remitting disorders and the transition from full-blown relapse to stability and recovery is a gradual process. In traditional crisis intervention literature this was anguished over interminably involving detailed speculations on the state of psychological defence mechanisms. In current teams the definition is ostensibly more concrete '...*would otherwise need hospitalization*'. In truth this is equally speculative – there is no external benchmark for knowing when a patient would need to be in hospital. It is always a complex clinical judgement based on risk, distress, and the practicalities of treatments.

Home treatment during a psychotic relapse

Sunita is 32 years old and lives with her parents and sister. She quit her university studies after a psychotic breakdown 2 years previously, but manages her job as a pharmacy assistant in the family shop. Her CMHT referred her to the CR/HT team after she had stopped taking her medication for 10 weeks and was becoming aggressive, disorganized, and forgetful (leaving the cooker on and lit cigarettes around). She was sleeping poorly and losing weight. Her consultant referred her at the point where he would otherwise have admitted her.

During the first week she was restless, agitated, extremely uncooperative, and very difficult to engage. She would not talk to members of the team and only took medication after a lot of persuasion. She received daily visits but these were restricted to medication management (she would not accept wider support or discussions) plus support to her family.

There was a slight improvement in the second week. Although she was still not engaging well she was not as uncommunicative as before, and she took her medicine with less persuasion. During this week there was the odd day without visits, although the family was phoned to confirm she had taken her tablets. There were no reports of her pestering her mother for cigarettes or being hostile. However during the visits that were made there was a noticeable softening – discussing worries she had, and even a request for us to bring some magazines next time.

During the third week Sunita became communicative, calm, and pleasant. She needed no persuasion to take her medicine, taking it as a matter of course. By the final week she had gained weight and was sleeping well. She was being visited every other day and had attended the outpatient department once. Her family felt confident to leave her alone for a weekend – unthinkable just a few weeks previously. During discharge planning meetings she talked about courses she wanted to attend and welcomed the transfer back to the CMHT. In total, she was in the care of the CR/HT team for 31 days.

Crisis Helpline **Initial Contact Sheet**

Date ..../..../....　　　　　　　　　　　　　Name ....

Time call received ....　　　　　Address ....

Time call ended ....　　　　　..............................

Helpline telephone Ref. Number ....　　　DOB ....

Type of call. Please circle as appropriate

| SILENT | NON-RELEVANT | WRONG NUMBER | INTOXICATED |
| INTERVENTION | PROFESSIONAL REFERRING TO | INFORMATION ONLY | ABUSIVE |

Was the Caller: Please answer all

Intoxicated　Y/N　　　　　Abusive　Y/N　　　　　　Regular caller　Y/N

Reason for call

Is there any evidence for, or has the client expressed any of the following

Self-harm?　Y/N　If yes how?

....

Violence to others?　　　Y/N　　　　　If yes towards whom? ....

Past psychiatric history?　　Y/N

Any current psychiatric interventions?　Y/N

Current medication?　　　　Y/N

If yes are they compliant?　Y/N

Are there any child protection issues?　　　　Y/N　　　　　If yes please give details

What immediate support is available?　(e.g. partner, family, friends) ....

....

Has the crisis affected regular lifestyle?　　Y/N　　　　　If yes how? ....

(e.g. sleep, appetite, anxiety, depression, motivation etc)　　　　　　.................................

....

Does the client require referral to:

Crisis Response Team	Y/N If yes please complete CRT referral form
Duty psychiatrist A&E	Y/N
Liaison nursing team	Y/N
Emergency services 999	Y/N
Emergency duty team/Approved social worker	Y/N

Does the client require referral to their own:

GP	Y/N
CPN	Y/N
Consultant	Y/N
Day care resource centre	Y/N
Care Manager	Y/N

Will the client make the referral for themselves?　　　Y/N

Will the client need the referral to be made on their behalf?　Y/N

Summary of action taken: (to include time and place of any onward referral)

Signed

Print name

Time/date

Fig. 6.2 Telephone helpline initial contact sheet

An alternative to hospital?

The history of psychiatry teaches us that we invariably underestimate the process of natural recovery. We attribute improvement to our treatments and keep patients in care longer than they need unless forced to do otherwise by external pressures (whether the closure of the mental hospital or a current bed shortage). CR/HT teams are only somewhat less vulnerable to this than the rest of us. Although most considered that crisis involvement should last 3–6 weeks (about equivalent to the length of a routine admission currently in the UK) all appear to keep patients considerably longer. About 3–6 months was more typical of the teams visited with the odd individual much longer.

A fairly cursory examination of capacity in CR/HT teams also quickly dispels the idea that they are restricted to patients who would otherwise be in hospital. The numbers simply do not stack up. What is true is that their primary task (that which gives the team its ethos and identity) is to provide intensive support and treatment to a small number of patients who would otherwise have to be admitted. The team will undoubtedly stay in contact with them longer than they would have needed to be in hospital. There is a 'halo' of patients who would, in fact, have been managed at home by the CMHT or AO team but have similar needs (for supervision, evening visits etc.) as those who would need immediate admission. CR/HT teams (like all other CMHTs) seem to use capacity and demand to inform decisions about who receives their services. These processes are reviewed below.

Team structure and staffing

Staffing

The policy implementation guide recommends a team size of about 14 full-time staff. It is proposed that such a team would provide for a population of about 150,000 (though clearly this will vary according to local circumstances) and have a caseload of between 20 and 30 patients at any one time. This is a fairly large CMHT. However, it would have difficulty functioning if much smaller as it has to operate extended hours and 7 days a week. CR/HT team staffing composition seems remarkably consistent.

Team leader

CR/HT teams draw heavily on assertive outreach team structure and process. Consequently they are lead by a team leader/manager who has a reduced caseload and whose tasks are predominantly running the team and providing supervision for the staff. The team manager can come from any of the key disciplines. Not surprisingly, given the staffing of CR/HT teams they are often nurses. Their role is outlined in more detail in Chapter 4.

Mental health nurses

Mental health nurses are the main professional group – usually constituting more than half the team – as medication management and delivery are core functions. Nurses also have an established role in providing direct personal care and are regularly judged to be the most tolerant and supportive of mental health staff. They usually come from CPN posts in generic CMHTs or from acute wards. There is a consensus that inpatient nurses transfer well to CR/HT teams.

'After all it's just like a ward in the patient's home.'

CR/HT teams really do have to operate a 'team approach' with shared tasks and, often, daily allocation of duties. This fits well with the ward experience, as does the task-centred and short-term focus of the teams.

Unique contribution of nurses

Although all CR/HT staff have expanded roles, some interventions around medication (e.g. giving depot injections) and much direct personal care cannot be shared with other disciplines. Consequently most teams treat the nurses as a discrete group when rostering shifts to ensure that there are always enough on. Similarly for on-call duties at least one of the on-call staff needs to be a nurse. The issues of gender and ethnic representation (see Chapter 4, Assertive outreach teams) are most relevant to the nurses in a CR/HT team, both because they are the most numerous group but also because of the intimate nature of the personal care they deliver. They are also the professional group with whom patients most commonly identify.

Medical staff

Most of the referrals to the team will be acutely ill and many will need consideration of admission under the Mental Health Act. Most will require careful prescribing and medication monitoring. Ready access to skilled medical input is essential. In practice all CR/HT teams have a full-time psychiatrist plus access on a sessional basis to a consultant psychiatrist.

Teams vary in how the psychiatrist operates but all consider them essential. Some teams strive to involve the psychiatrist as much as possible in all assessments. Others only call on the psychiatrist when the patient has been accepted onto the team and there is a clinical need. There may be considerable variation in local practice (even within the same Trust) about whether or not the team takes on full consultant and CPA responsibility.

Given such wide variation in practice it would be unhelpful to describe the roles and responsibilities of the doctor in any detail – time will tell which models work best. The core activities of the doctor in the team are, however, fairly consistent and also fairly traditional. They are responsible for assessments, diagnosis, and monitoring of mental state, and for prescribing. They are inevitably involved in decisions about potential admissions (a significant proportion of CR/HT patients are admitted, though hopefully for shortened stays), particularly those involving the Mental Health Act.

On-call availability

The policy implementation guide stresses 24-hour access to senior psychiatrists able to do home visits. In practice this is neither happening nor necessary (see below 'Hours of Operation'). Most services use the local 24-hour duty psychiatrist who is usually available for A&E and possibly for inpatient back-up. This is sensible and works well. However, much of the current writing on the topic implies that the CR/HT team should have its *own exclusive* 24-hour on-call doctor. Striving for such a uniform, comprehensive service at night has little to recommend it either in theory or in practice. A slavish adherence to it has already been responsible for confusion in the AO literature and, in part, for the demise of one otherwise excellent community psychiatry development (Stefansson and Cullberg 1986). One service has a shared duty doctor rota solely for assertive outreach, crisis, and continuing care teams, which increases the chances of the duty doctor having good knowledge of team principles and possibly of the patients (Wood and Carr 1998).

Social workers

Social workers are generally core members of CR/HT teams. Their systems and family approach to problems are highly appropriate for dealing with crises and mobilizing local resources to support relapsing individuals. A highly developed understanding of local resources, familiarity with the social services emergency staff, plus access to emergency funding and, if need be, accommodation are specific benefits they bring to the team.

Independence of ASW

Some teams rely on their social worker to act as their ASW whereas others prefer to keep this function separate. Most of the patients who are going to need compulsory treatment will be known to the routine services. Some teams consider it best practice to avoid using their own social worker as ASW because of concerns over independence. Others simply consider it safer to rely on the duty system as no team can always ensure it has an ASW available.

Traditional problems around social workers integrating into CMHTs (such as duplicate note keeping and parallel lines of accountability) are rapidly disappearing with the development of Health and Social Care Trusts. None of CR/HT teams visited reported any major problems with integration of their social worker colleagues.

Occupational therapists and clinical psychologists

Occupational therapists

Many teams have occupational therapists as staff. They take part in the generic working of the team but, not surprisingly, bring a strong emphasis to the preservation of individual functioning, and the organization of activities and time-tables for both patient and family. This sophisticated approach to structuring time is highly appreciated by crisis patients and their families.

A sense of helplessness is common in a crisis. It can result in abandoning even those functions that the patient or family could still manage, and which, if maintained, might reduce some of the sense of collapse and failure. For instance, although a patient is too ill to work, with encouragement and support they could still pick up the children from school, do some simple shopping or the laundry. Occupational therapists are alert to just how important exercising competence is for self-esteem. Just when other team members may suggest ignoring family duties for the time being when the patient is too distressed the OT's professional commitment to supporting autonomy can provide a healthy counterbalance.

Clinical psychologists

None of the teams visited had a clinical psychologist fully integrated though some did have sessional input and most had access. Most staff in CR/HT teams think that a clinical psychologist on the team would be '*a good thing*'. However, unlike Early intervention teams, there is no clarity about what their specific role would be. Complex psychological interventions are unlikely to loom large in a CR/HT team. These are more likely to be initiated by the routine services when the crisis is over.

Clinical psychologists and occupational therapists on all CMHTs perform a vital task of keeping the intellectual framework of the team broad. They benefit by not having statutory roles in the team in the way the doctors, nurses, and social workers all do. The pressure to adopt a limited medical approach is probably greater in the CR/HT team than any of the other CMHTs because they are continually dealing with acutely ill patients ('*like a ward in the community*'). Clinical psychologists and occupational therapists, quite apart from their specific inputs, keep the team open minded, which is no small contribution.

Mental health support workers

Mental health support workers work particularly well in CR/HT teams and are highly valued by the professional staff. The support/therapy balance inclines significantly more towards support in these teams compared to other CMHTs. The CR/HT team provides monitoring, direct care, and encouragement through the crisis – very much as ward staff or an extended family would. Medicines take time to work and during this time the patient and family are distressed, and the situation volatile. Treatments cannot simply be intensified or speeded up. There is no added value in giving medicines 4 times a day rather than 2, counselling sessions require time for absorption and consolidation. What the patient and carers need is company and support while the treatments take effect.

Support and direct help

Mental health support workers deal better than professionals with much of this support and direct help. They are not handicapped by professional expectations and a sense that they are not doing what they were trained for, or that others need their skills more (as doctors and nurses so often do). Their jargon-free, practical approach is a real asset. Assisting with, or even doing, the daily chores can relieve an overwhelming burden for those in crisis and permit them to use their energies to get well. Obviously this has to be balanced with autonomy as discussed above. It is rare, however, for a family in crisis not to benefit when offered direct help and support.

As with all CMHTs the mental health support workers should be chosen, as far as possible, to reflect the characteristics of the local population. Such matching aids engagement and trust and also gives insight into idiosyncratic local solutions to problems:

A young Turkish man arrived in A&E in a highly disorganized and distraught state. He was convinced that his family wanted to kill him because they had found out that he was homosexual and felt that it would disgrace them. His English was excellent (he moved here when he was 11 years old) and it was clear that he was also experiencing somatic hallucinations and demonstrating thought disorder. His family came to A&E and were very keen for him not to be admitted to hospital. They were also confused and distressed and convinced that his problems were due to drug abuse.

He was willing to return home where he was initially visited twice a day and took antipsychotic medication. Although things settled for the first couple of days both he and his family began to become increasingly wound up, and there were two quite worrying outbursts. He adamantly refused respite in the crisis house or in a B&B as he was now convinced that people hated him for being Turkish and would abuse him there. The team was concerned that the risk to his disabled father was escalating and that he might have to be admitted.

The team's Turkish support worker had spent many hours with the family, comforting and reassuring the mother and distracting and occupying the patient by playing backgammon. When admission was being discussed he mentioned a Turkish widow in the next borough who took only Turkish lodgers. He knew her well and thought she would take the patient for a short time as long as he visited regularly. The patient liked the house and the landlady, felt safe in an all-Turkish environment and settled there for over a week while his delusions started to recede and he could return to his family.

Many teams earmark a proportion of the mental health support worker posts for users and this seems to work as well in CR/HT teams as others – i.e. very well indeed.

Hours of operation and shift working

Rapid accessibility is the hallmark of the CR/HT team so they operate 7 days a week with some form of 24-hour service. Some teams treat all 7 days the same with a shift system rostered equally throughout the week. Some (like most AO and EIS teams) have a reduced availability at the weekend. There are never less than two staff on at any given time.

In some well functioning services (where CMHTs offer effective crisis provision to their own patients during "office hours") CR/HT teams concentrate their resources on evenings and weekends. Doctors are not rostered for shifts. Medical staff work office hours (though individuals are often very flexible) and the emergency service (whether this was operated from within the team or, more often, from the local routine service provision) provides medical input for evenings and weekends.

North Birmingham Ladywood team:

6 staff on the early shift	(09.00–17.00)
2 staff on the late shift	(13.00–21.00). Late shift staff on-call overnight

South Islington team:

4 staff on the early shift	(08.30–16.30)
4 staff on the late shift	(14.00–22.00) Two of late shift on-call overnight

Shifts

Most CR/HT teams operate a shift system. This means that the team is fully operational at least 12 hours a day, usually from 8.00am to 9.00pm. How shifts are organized differs. Here are two examples:

Review and handover meetings

Daily reviews

Daily review meetings to start the day are an essential aspect of CR/HT teams because of the high level of team working and the need to share out tasks on a daily basis. These meetings are similar to AO 'handovers' (with each patient being mentioned by name) but are more detailed in their allocation of tasks. Early morning telephone calls are very common and are dealt with at this meeting. Experienced A&E doctors often deal with crises, sending the patient home in the night having promised a visit from the CR/HT team the next day. Rather than wake the duty worker they either leave a message on the answerphone or ring as they are going off duty.

The white board

Usually all the patients' names are on a white board and each identified task or visit is written up along with the time and who is responsible for it. Because there are usually only 10–20 patients who need detailed consideration the meeting still only takes about 30 minutes (Ladywood schedules 60 minutes). It may be a little longer on Monday when everyone is catching up. Not every patient is mentioned at every meeting (see 'zoning' below).

Daily handovers

Effective shift working requires regular and efficient handing over of information. The daily handover meeting is very similar to what happens on admission wards. There are variations in how it can be conducted and in the two teams above it is quite different.

Crisis Team Daily Planning Board

Name	Sector	Crisis Co-ordinator	Visits	Diary	Today 12.12.02	Staff Member
JK	D	Jemma C	Twice daily	CPA on 23rd Dec 2pm. Review by doctor and care co-ordinator on Weds 14.12.02	HV 9am with medication. HV 8pm for support to carers and make arrangements for tomorrow's visits	Debbie M + Nina L
FG	E	Tina J	Daily	Meds due 19th Dec. Book interpreter for next week's visit	HV tonight with interpreter and Child and Family Social Worker	Matt W + June S
LV	E	Ola A	Twice daily	Ask Caroline G to ring Med Sec. Recently discharged from hospital. P/C family for support	HV this pm. Check if heating is on? And what is in the fridge?	Jemma C
NA	D	Kofi A	Daily	Housing have crime number re harrassment. Ring Police 22.12 for update	HV as late as possible for support. Assess noise in flat. Book CT scan. P/C medical foundation	Matt W + June S
CD	D	Auxilia R	Daily	Discuss risk assessment with consultant. Blood results due back 15.12	HV this afternoon with care co-ordinator to prepare for discharge back to CMHT	Nina L
SS	D	Carlton R	Daily	Vickie K to visit on 15.12 to discuss referral to Irish Support Group	Visit am to see family and to give information and support re diagnosis	Carlton R + Auxilia R
GK	E	Montse G	Twice daily	Refer to CMHT for long term follow-up	HV am. Needs help to fill in benefit forms. HV pm. Can we do some shopping with GK (use petty cash)	Auxilia R + Meghan G

In the Ladywood team all the early shift aim to come back to base at 1pm to handover to all of the late shift. Everyone is present and after the meeting they can go off and do more visits. In the South Islington team, however it is the team leader who is responsible for the handover in the middle of the day to the late shift. They have decided that bringing all the team back at 2pm is too disruptive and so the team leader (having been at the morning review meeting) is able to brief the late shift. Some teams aim for a very brief 'signing off' meeting at about 4.30pm. This is mainly for safety issues.

In depth reviews

Although there appears to be no consistency about whether or not CR/HT teams take CPA responsibility (as with variation in consultant responsibility) there is still a need for the team to review patients in detail, beyond the regular morning and handover meetings. Most teams identify a session a week when special problems can receive more reflective consideration. This is usually a meeting where sessional staff (e.g. clinical psychologist, consultant psychiatrist) are present. Carving out time to think without having to respond immediately to a current pressure is particularly important for CR/HT teams who otherwise can be caught up in a whirl. As with all other CMHTs this is a time when risk assessments, structured mental state assessments, or needs assessments can be discussed and presented. Even if the team does not have CPA responsibility, careful and comprehensive documentation is always required and this meeting gives the opportunity to review and amend it.

Referrals and assessments

CR/HT teams have a high volume of referral and throughput. Assessments of new patients is a significant part of their work and there is no expectation that all patients assessed will be taken on for care. Both the Ladywood team and the South Islington teams averaged about 8–10 referrals a week, which is similar to that in urban CMHTs (Burns *et al.* 1993*a*). About 75% of referrals do not suffer from a psychotic illness (again similar to CMHTs) although those taken on for care are more likely to do so. The South Islington team estimated that they remained involved beyond assessment in about two-thirds of referrals.

Balancing focus with access

Although the Policy Implementation guide has a long list of exclusions it is clear that most teams operate a fairly tolerant approach to assessment. This is not surprising as it is often remarkably difficult to be sure what the problem is until you see the patient – especially if they are new to the service and distressed. Ladywood had thought through this issue carefully and made a policy decision not to filter referrals – 'a team that does not say no'. South Islington, on the other hand, often discussed potential referrals on the phone and rerouted a steady, though uncertain, proportion. Differences in approach will reflect the volume of referrals and familiarity with local referrers. As with any team, too rigid an insistence on referral criteria diminishes its value (see Chapter 3).

The assessment process

CR/HT teams devote considerable time and thought to the assessment process, often breaking it down into several stages.

1. Pre-assessment phase.
2. Assessment phase.
3. Planning phase.

Pre-assessment phase

The referral form is utilized to collect as much information from available sources as possible before undertaking the assessment. This is an active process with staff taking responsibility to seek information – not just being passive recipients ('make three telephone calls before you go', 'decide on who will go and what needs to be taken').

Assessment phase

The individual is encouraged to talk at length 'there is no hurry'. This can obviously be an intensive experience and staff anticipate tolerating anger and distress. The assessment aims at more than just coming to a decision about the problem and also aims for the establishment of some positive relationship with the patient.

Planning phase

This emphasizes involving the wider social network wherever possible. It includes making sure that everyone knows of the team's availability and what it can do. Management options are formulated and discussed and the consequences of these discussed. Active listening and strengthening the relationship continues throughout this phase. Addressing basic survival needs (e.g. food, electricity) is generally thought of as part of the planning phase.

The implementation plan

As with assessment it is common to structure the implementation plan developed at that assessment.

1. Immediate implementation.
2. Medium term implementation.
3. Final stage of implementation.

Immediate implementation

This phase focuses on explaining the treatment plan so that everyone is clear about what is involved and what to do. Basic needs such as food, finance, and accommodation will dominate this phase. Immediate problems are addressed so that the patient and those directly involved can be sufficiently settled to get a decent night's sleep. The time of the next visit is arranged – it is not enough simply to say 'someone will be around tomorrow'.

Medium term implementation

This spans the period of frequent visiting (several times a week or even daily and more) when treatments are being introduced and mental state is being carefully monitored. Addressing practical problems remains high on the agenda and family and friends may need extensive attention and reassurance. This is a time when the needs identified at the first assessment are reconsidered and updated and hopefully treatment effects noted.

Final stage implementation

Generally this is when the crisis is resolved and visits reduced to weekly or even less. Introduction to the CMHT key-worker, if appropriate, takes place then. A debriefing is particularly valuable – 'what happened and caused all that? What did we both learn from it that we can use again if need be?'

Who makes the referrals?

Between a third and a half of referrals come from CMHTs, the rest from A&E and GPs. Whether AO and EIS teams refer varies enormously, depending on local arrangements and also whether or not they have their own beds. AO and EIS teams may make specific referrals for 'partial or shared treatment' (see below). Most referrals are by telephone. Figure 6.3 is an example of a crisis team's referral form. The added value of these referral forms in audit and service planning is outlined in Chapter 2.

About 50% of referrals are new to the team – the other 50% are rereferrals of relapsing patients. Not surprisingly rereferrals (and appropriate referrals that are taken on for care) are more common from CMHTs who soon form a clear and accurate assessment of what the CR/HT team can offer. Inappropriate referrals (notably intoxicated individuals) are most likely from A&E and from GP deputising services where the referrer has never met the patient before. It is important for teams to be realistic about this and not get too precious.

Who conducts sssessments?

Joint assessments for unknown patients

Most teams aim to have a joint assessment of any patient who is unknown to them. Two members of staff conduct the assessment and report back. In Ladywood a psychiatrist is always involved in the assessment during office hours whereas in South Islington this is not usual. Here the psychiatrist is called in after the first assessment if it is thought that prescribing will be necessary, or if the case is complex. Obviously a psychiatrist is also involved if the assessment includes a decision about use of the Mental Health Act.

These two high profile teams have evolved their own systems and there is no information about how representative these approaches are, nor of their relative merits. Most of the patients will have had a psychiatric assessment before referral so the

| **Crisis Resolution Team** |
| **Referral Form** |

| Date & Time: | Staff Member: |
| .... |

Title:	Surname:	Forename:
Address:		
	Post Code:	Sector D/E
	DOB:	Gender: M/F
Phone: Home		
Work		
Single	Married/Cohab	Ethnic Origin:	
Widowed	Divorced/Sep	Language	Int. Req'd Yes ❑ No ❑

Next Kin: Relationship:
Addr
Tel:

GP: Addr

Tel: Code:

Keyworker:

Tel:

Referred by:	CPA Exists: Yes ❑ No ❑
	Paid Emp: Yes ❑ No ❑
	No of Admission: 1 ❑ 2 ❑ 3 ❑ 4 ❑
	(*Last 12 Mths*)
Tel:	
Reason for referral	

Continue overleaf if necessary

Referrer's expectation of team: (*could resolution be more appropriately provided by other services?*)

Psych history? Nil ❑   Past ❑   Current ❑   Current diagnosis:

Previous contact with CRT: Yes ❑   No ❑

Current Meds:

Recreational drug use?

Other services involved:

| Action: (incl. date and time) | Not appropriate for CRT (tick) ❑ |

First face to face contact   Date: Time:

Where assessed: Home ❑   Office ❑   A&E ❑   Ward ❑   Police ❑   CMHT ❑   Other ❑

Fig. 6.3 Crisis Resolution/Home Treatment Team Referral Form

increasing emphasis on medical involvement in CMHT new patient assessments (Department of Health 2002) may be less relevant.

In the 50% of referrals already known to the team it may be acceptable for the assessment to be conducted by one team member during routine working hours.

If there are concerns about safety (and always with new patients) two members conduct the assessment. If in doubt this needs to be agreed with the team manager. Because of the high frequency of contact it is quite possible for assessments to be prolonged, involving two or three visits, though this is not common.

Caseload management

The policy implementation guide recommends that the CR/HT team is structured as a AO team to reflect high staffing and low caseloads. In practice most CR/HT teams reflect the caseload management style of EIS teams with a zoning system (see Chapter 5). Patients have a named worker (essentially a key worker) but the balance between care co-ordination and care provision is quite different to that in either AO or EIS. In the CR/HT team the emphasis really is on co-ordination as patients are visited by several team members – sometimes on the same day. Continuity of care at this level of intensity is simply not possible at an individual level.

Composition of caseload

It has proved difficult to gain a clear picture of the caseload composition of CR/HT teams. Staff remember difficult patients such as those with severe mania or very disturbed psychotic patients. As with all CMHTs examination of the figures usually demonstrates these to be a smaller proportion than believed. The caseload from one long-established team was:

- Psychosis   35%
- Affective disorder (bipolar, depression and relationship problems)   30%
- Personality disorder/situational crisis   20%
- Alcohol and drug abuse   15%

These are revealing and honest figures and represent the reality rather than the rhetoric of CR/HT teams. Around half will be suffering from a psychotic disorder and probably not much more than half will really fit the bill of the current guidance (Department of Health 2001). This patient mix does, however, allow for coherent and meaningful practice and there is little reason to believe that these patients are not significantly disabled by their illnesses and in need of intensive care.

Contact frequency and distribution

Frequency

The core target group of patients – those who would otherwise be in hospital – receive daily visits and often more than once a day for the first few days of their care. Few continue at frequencies in excess of once a day for more than a week or so – there are probably not more than 3–5 patients on multiple visits at any time in a team. Visits can, however, be very extended and often staff will stay with patients for several hours in the beginning (see mental health support worker above). In exceptionally rare circumstances patients have received up to 4 visits a day.

TP is a 27-year-old woman with a 3-month-old son. She had post-natal depression and was previously treated in hospital. There were also ongoing relationship problems with her partner. Once discharged, she did not comply with her medication and soon started to deteriorate. Her partner wanted to take the little boy away, saying she was not capable of looking after him. The emergency duty social worker assessed her with a view to readmission. TP would not go into hospital, believing that her partner would take the child permanently away from her. The Social worker had either to admit her on section or arrange additional support for her and the child through the CR/HT team and decided on the latter.

The Home Treatment team visited TP twice daily to monitor her mental health, ensure compliance with medication, and provide support.

They found that the relationship problem was partly due to beliefs and stigma about mental health in the partner's culture. So he was educated about mental illness and caring. He was persuaded to give TP more physical support with housework, which he readily did.

The intervention proved to be surprisingly effective and smooth. A striking improvement was seen within a week of her restarting medication and visits were down to daily by the end of the second week. TP's care co-ordinator also arranged home help for her.

Telephone contact

Most teams have high levels of telephone contact with patients. A late night call to ensure the patient is settled can be reassuring for all concerned. Reminders to take medicines can be by phone when patients no longer need intensive monitoring. The use of text messaging is increasing. This is a form of communication welcomed by younger patients (and staff) and has the advantage of being less public and intrusive than a voice call.

Night visits

Scheduled visits after 9.00pm were rare in teams visited. Overall about 70–75% of all contacts were during 'regular shift hours'. After 9.00pm contacts were generally restricted to assessments. Most teams had anticipated having to stay overnight with patients or visit them often at home in the night but this had simply not been the case. The pattern generally was that one of the two on-call staff was fairly active up to about midnight – usually on the telephone or in A&E. Getting out of bed after that was rare. The South Islington team had recorded 15 'call-outs' after midnight over a six-month period – about one every two weeks. In Ladywood the team conducted about 10% of their visits between and 11.00pm–2.00am and virtually none after that. On the other hand it is a rare evening shift with no work. In Ladywood the on-call nurses conducted an assessment on average each second night. In a recent four-week audit, however, there were only three nights with no calls at all for the team.

Night visits are almost entirely assessments and always in places of safety such as A&E or occasionally police stations. *Teams do not visit patients in their homes at night* despite the widely held belief that this is their aim. Both on-call staff attend for night visits and these are usually when the A&E psychiatrist considers that an admission is indicated. In Ladywood the CR/HT team calls their own medic to this assessment but this is not the case in South Islington. South Islington estimated that about half of the night assessments were admitted but this was lower in Ladywood. In the other half the CR/HT team identified alternatives – often taking the patient home after suitable medication and with plans for prompt follow up.

On-call arrangements

Twenty-four-hour availability in most teams is provided by staff on-call from home. Some services use pagers and others mobile phones; some have a first and second on-call, some simply two equally on-call. Doctors are accessed through varying duty-rotas. Careful management of on-call duties is a tricky business. If there is nothing to do staff get bored and dissatisfied, if there is too much to do then it can become too expensive and undermine the service. In the two teams highlighted in this chapter staff were generally very satisfied with on-call arrangements and were paid about 20 hours overtime per month per individual. The 9.00–12.00pm period was often used to catch up with paperwork while dealing with calls in the office before going home.

Partial or shared treatment 'top-up work'

Where AO or CMHT teams are running well they may often provide a passable home treatment function themselves. Certainly all AO teams should be able to visit patients once or twice daily for extended periods and there are many CMHTs who pride themselves on being able to support the occasional patient with daily visits for short periods. CMHTs may call on the CR/HT to augment this input by, for instance, providing visits at the weekend. This is referred to as 'top-up' work in North Birmingham, augmenting the function of the CMHT. In this situation the CR/HT team does not take over the patient but works in a supporting role to the CMHT.

The AO team or CMHT might ask the CR/HT team to visit in the evenings for a few days, perhaps to supervise medication or ensure that the patient is settling down. This is generally thought to be an excellent use of CR/HT team skills and resources. It is rewarding to staff and particularly helpful in fostering good relations with other teams. These patients are registered on the white board and discussed (as 'green' patients) at handovers but usually the notes remain with the CMHT or AO team. Prioritizing this support function rather than an independent and gatekeeping role as the main purpose of the CR/HT team is being explored in several services.

Zoning

Most teams run with more than the recommended 20–30 patients on their caseloads. about 35–40 is more common and sometimes this is exceeded for periods. These higher caseloads reflect difficulties in handing on (see below) rather than choice, often with several patients being maintained on low-frequency contact while awaiting transfer. This is managed by zoning (see Chapter 5). Zoning thresholds in CR/HT teams reflect their different contact frequency compared to EIS teams:

- Red   Contact daily and above.
- Amber   Contact 2–3 times a week.
- Green   Contact weekly and below.

Red and Amber patients are mentioned at every handover but Green patients only discussed intermittently – usually at the weekly in-depth reviews

Liaison and handover

It will be clear from what has been written about the remit of different CR/HT teams that there is no uniform pattern of how they relate to the services around them. At one extreme the team takes full responsibility for all aspects of their patients' care (consultant and CPA responsibility is transferred and it manages its own beds). For such teams liaison is fairly uncomplicated and consists mainly of arranging joint handover meetings for individual patients when they are moving on to the CMHT or AO team.

If consultant responsibility does not transfer fully (and certainly if inpatient care is retained by the referring team) then mutually acceptable liaison arrangements need to be agreed upon and maintained. As emphasized in Chapters 4 and 5 it is more important that liaison and transfer arrangements are mutually agreed, crystal clear, and written down than the details of what they are. Almost any arrangement will work provided all parties have genuinely agreed on it and are committed to it.

Inpatient liaison

Team members may visit inpatients if under the care of the CMHT so that they can assist with early discharge planning. It is not uncommon for a patient to be admitted from the CR/HT team and to be temporarily returned to that team at discharge while they stabilize before being finally transferred back to the CMHT. Liaison with the ward will vary depending mainly on how many teams the CR/HT team relates to. The visiting may be personalized if the team only deals with a single CMHT (named workers visit 'their' patients). On the other hand if they regularly relate to several teams then a designated link worker serves each CMHT or ward. Clinical judgement is exercised and the CR/HT team does not necessarily have to remain involved with inpatients, and usually will only be involved with a minority anticipated to have very short admissions and needing CR/HT involvement on discharge.

Liaison meetings with CMHTs

Where responsibilities (e.g. consultant or CPA responsibility) continue to be shared between the CR/HT team and the referring team, then a robust and practical liaison system is essential. The commonest is for a consistent CR/HT link worker to attend the team meetings each week. Usually the CMHT will ensure that the relevant patients are discussed early in the meeting so that the link worker's time is used efficiently. As well as co-ordinating care these meetings are invaluable for taking the temperature between the teams and smoothing out any tensions that may arise. Misunderstandings and disagreements about relative roles in the care of difficult patients are inevitable, even in the best run services. Time spent on liaison and fostering decent working relationships is always time well spent.

Handing back

Once the crisis is over and the patient is no longer at risk of imminent admission they go back to the referring team or (if they are new to the service) are referred on to the appropriate one. That is how it is supposed to happen and often does. But not always. For some patients the resolution of the crisis may mean that they can be discharged back to their GP or they may even refuse further contact. Typically with such patients the CR/HT team may work slightly longer with them to ensure that all loose ends are tied up.

Where patients have come from one of the secondary care teams and are known to the service then CR/HT teams would expect to transfer back when contact is down to once a week or certainly every two weeks. Transfer back to AO and EIS services may occur at a higher contact frequency as these teams would be expected to be able to maintain that input. Handover is usually by joint working across the two teams.

Disagreements

Inevitably there will be disagreements about whether or not a patient is ready for transfer. Often the receiving team will think the patient is still not well enough. Sometimes this is really a thinly disguised 'respite' for the routine team (just as admission can be). It is important for CR/HT teams to recognize that this is both inevitable and, in many ways, healthy. GPs have long recognized that a temporary referral to secondary services can give them a breather and enable them to avoid becoming too burnt out with difficult and intractable patients.

Situations do, however, arise when the appropriate team simply refuses to take the patient and the CR/HT team manager and consultant may have to bring real pressure to bear. If not the team can become silted up and unable to discharge its duties, and patients may become trapped in a team that is not appropriate for their long-term needs.

Time and energy spent arguing back and forth around handovers is a significant drain on CR/HT team resources (and indeed of the resisting team also). There seems to be no easy solution to it – drawing up guidelines does not help much, as the issues are invariably subjective judgements about severity. Every boundary in mental health care introduces a 'transaction cost' which is the price that has to be paid for increasing specialization. It is not trivial and needs to be part of decision-making about local team structures.

Gatekeeping and inpatient care

Benefits of routine gatekeeping

The policy implementation guide (Department of Health 2001) emphasizes the gatekeeping function of the CR/HT team, proposing that all admissions should go through it whether from CMHT, EIS, or AO teams. This is seen as essential if bed occupancy is to be reduced but also if the other teams are to acquire an understanding of what the CR/HT team can offer. If all the admissions are not assessed by the CR/HT team then other teams will continue to make their traditional assumptions about thresholds for admission. They will not learn how the CR/HT team can provide alternatives and thereby alter that threshold. This is a compelling case.

Resistance to routine gatekeeping

These are new teams and until other staff have experience of what they have to offer then they may be reluctant to refer to them. New teams inevitably cause some resentment and it is not unlikely that the established teams may be sceptical:

> I've known her for years. She always needs to come in when she gets like this and if kept out things just get worse. I've got a good relationship with her and her family. What do the crisis team think they can do that I can't?

While the logic behind gatekeeping is clear, and certainly makes sense as a way of mutual education, it is often resented. None of the current teams felt that it always worked. In particular they found it difficult to convince consultant psychiatrists who were in the process of admitting to their own team's beds. Not all teams will go along with this gatekeeping role and their position is equally understandable.

There is good evidence from clinical practice that bed management is generally better when continuity of responsibility is unbroken. There are no 'perverse incentives' attached to admission in getting away from a difficult problem. Studies of suicide rates in discharged patients indicate that transfer of responsibility between teams raises the risk (Appleby *et al.* 1999). Lastly the imperative to reduce inpatient care may be less pressing in well-functioning services with good bed management. For them the rationale for gatekeeping is less convincing and consequently the downsides of discontinuity of care and the time taken to effect transfers less acceptable.

Inpatient care

CR/HT teams do not take responsibility for acute ward inpatients although some have a range of respite alternatives. These can be beds in a crisis centre or a respite house (as in EIS, see Chapter 5). One team had a designated short-term bed on a rehabilitation ward. Most teams acquire a set of Bed and Breakfast establishments they work closely with for urgent short-term respite. While the CR/HT team relinquishes responsibility to the routine team when the patient is admitted they often maintain contact if the admission is likely to be brief (see above) and they are going to be involved in reintegration.

Notes and documentation

Most Trusts have global policies about notes and the CR/HT team will usually be bound by this. If there is a single set of notes the CR/HT team uses them, but in some cases they may raise their own set of notes (which are reused with subsequent further contacts). This approach certainly seems to work better – the notes are focused around the special practices of the team and much more manageable. Completing a detailed summary on discharge that goes into the patient's main notes ensures that the routine team is well informed and helps reduce the burgeoning expansion of notes (often running into several volumes for some SMI patients).

Documentation

Some form of brief referral form is particularly useful in CR/HT teams. This is filled out by the staff member who takes the call. It helps give the team an overview of its work and also is an immediately available guide to the problem for workers in the first couple of days before a more detailed history is recorded. Otherwise documentation is very like that in AO teams (see Chapter 4) with a clear need to have risk assessment and some form of care plan (whether or not it is part of CPA) recorded. Contingency plans are generally vestigial in CR/HT teams as they are in such close contact with their patients.

Dispensing and medication management

Enhanced role in prescribing and dispensing

CR/HT teams usually take more direct control over medication than other CMHTs. The approach reflects that of an inpatient unit. Patients have a drug card just as they would when inpatients so that changes can be made frequently and clearly. Drugs are prescribed by the team (in these acute situations shared care with the GP would be clumsy and risky) and often dispensed by the team. This works best if the team has a well-stocked drug cupboard and can (against the prescription) make up packs of daily or weekly drugs which are delivered directly to the patient. The use of dosette boxes is common and nurses on the team fill these. Taking the medication will often be directly supervised by team members.

Current dispensing legislation and local policies

The current legislation on drug dispensing in the UK is unclear. The common belief that dispensing can only be done by a pharmacist appears not to be the case and trained nursing staff can dispense (just as they would on a ward). The difference here is that they may be dispensing for several days. What is important is that the procedures are carefully worked out to ensure consistency and adequate checking, and that there is a written drug dispensing and administration policy that is agreed with the Trust.

On-call bag

As part of this active medication management approach most teams have an emergency bag which they take on new assessments. This will contain a selection of common medications (antipsychotics, benzodiazepines, antidepressants, and anticonvulsants) which can be used on the spot when prescribed by the doctor present (either the team's own doctor or the A&E or duty psychiatrist). A selection of empty bottles and labels allows a few days' doses to be individually arranged and left with the patient and family. Having such a bag is a godsend. The ability to prescribe there and then (perhaps a sleeping tablet and an antipsychotic), and then wait an hour or so until the patient begins to wind down means that they can often be safely taken home and settled down till the next morning when they can be visited.

The on-call bag usually contains a range of essential items in addition to the medicines and first-aid requirements:

Contents of an on-call bag

- A range of commonly required medicines – oral and IM.
- Copies of information leaflets, both about the service and common problems and drugs, are very useful to leave with patients and relatives.
- Some petty cash – a few pounds to buy essential groceries and feed the electricity meter can make the difference between remaining at home and having to be admitted.
- A list of essential telephone numbers including contact details for respite beds and short notes on which B&Bs the team uses and what they can deal with.
- Last, but not least, a torch and panic alarm for safety.

Using the ward, day hospitals, and day centres

Although the team aims to treat patients in their own homes and neighbourhoods it can sometimes be essential to obtain periods of respite for family members. A team member staying with the patient allows the family member to go out for a time. However, they may need time in their own home to get on with things or to rest without the patient being there.

Value of flexible 'guesting'

In such circumstances a flexible relationship with a ward or day facility which is willing to accommodate the patient for a few hours now and then works well. This is particularly so for hypomaniac or importunate, anxious patients who make relentless demands on their families. To work this has to be a flexible 'guesting' relationship and is quite different to the routine use of day hospitals or day centres. Usually the team members are responsible for bringing the patient to the ward and picking them up afterwards. Popping in while they are there also shows willingness and will increase the likelihood that the ward or day hospital will cooperate.

Specialist skills

CR/HT teams attract individuals who like the *'buzz'* of an active, task-centred approach. To be successful they need to be tolerant, well trained, good communicators, and clear thinking. It is difficult to identify specific techniques or skills that are unique to this approach, which seems to be a blend of CMHT and inpatient practices. More attention is needed than in most other teams to internal liaison, and maintaining clarity around exactly who is doing what. Care to avoid accidental duplication of medication doses and attention to safety checks on visits require a clear thinking, alert approach.

Social systems theory

The South Islington team has recently become influenced by the work of Paul Pollack and is trying to exploit the crisis situation by including as wide a range of family members and neighbours as possible in assessment and problem-solving meetings. They have found this valuable in widening their perspectives when trying to understand the crisis and it has yielded novel and unexpected solutions on several occasions. Like AO teams CR/HT teams have had to grapple with the issues of confidentiality but generally operate with the assumption that the crisis is usually public knowledge to neighbours and family. Patients are asked if they agree to these larger groupings. However, a culture of acknowledging the wider impact of the crisis is clear to all involved and, in some measure, invites the answer 'yes'.

Conclusions

CR/HT teams are probably the most varied of the new teams in how they relate to surrounding services. Their practice, however, is impressively consistent. They aim to combine the best of practice from a generic CMHT and a good inpatient ward and their unique contribution comes not so much from specific interventions as from their style of operating. Their strength is in their rapid availability and wide access – much more accepting than the policy implementation guide would have us believe.

Misunderstandings

CR/HT are also probably the most misunderstood of the new teams. This arises from two persistently repeated and misleading beliefs. The first is that they only deal with patients who would otherwise be in hospital. The second is that assessments of new patients are conducted in their homes at night. These two propositions are far from the truth and are responsible for much of the resistance to, and problems with, their development. Well-functioning services can see the overall advantages of a CR/HT team operating in their support. However, they may resist them because of the perceived impracticality and wastefulness which reflect these perpetuated misconceptions. If local bed management is good the reductions in admissions claimed will, rightly, be viewed sceptically and convincing evidence demanded.

The preoccupation with the merits or otherwise of gatekeeping and reduction in admissions, and the safety and necessity of nocturnal home visits often obscures the real advantages that such a service can, and does, bring.

Identifying component functions

As with AO teams the task is to look beyond the rhetoric and decide *what functions* such a team can fulfil that current services cannot. A broader, less hurried assessment of potential admissions with a clear focus on the social network stands out. Along with this is the ability to strengthen the support offered (particularly in evenings and at weekends) to patients teetering on the brink of admission.

We know that patients would rather be managed at home if it can be arranged and CR/HT teams have evolved impressive ways of providing necessary support. A reduction in the use of the Mental Health Act is an important benefit of this alternative. Being able to take a patient home and visit them promptly and regularly avoids having to admit them compulsorily if they can accept treatment. Without such a facility it may simply not be safe.

Disentangling the procedures from the structural issues (which are bound up with broader conflicting ideologies) is the way forward. Once we know better what the effective ingredients are in crisis work and home treatment we can examine the various models of providing it and find out what works and where.

CHAPTER 7

Highly specialized teams

The teams outlined so far in this book serve 'adults of working age'. They are, essentially, *different structures* for meeting the range of patient needs, rather than for meeting the needs of *different groups* of patients. This chapter will briefly overview how some of the more specialized teams (teams which are targeted on specific patient groups) adapt to these models. Many of the team structures and practices are remarkably similar (as, of course, are many of the patient needs) so it would be repetitive and unhelpful to describe them in great detail. Attention will be drawn to major differences that are common in them. It also goes without saying that they vary between themselves as do good teams based on any model.

The most numerous of these teams are those for children and adolescents and those for older patients. It is not possible to run comprehensive services without these teams operating within the same local provision as the adult teams described earlier. Beyond these age-related teams there is a second group of highly specialized teams which (although also important for providing a comprehensive service) may not be provided at the same local level. They may be provided across larger and variable catchment areas. Examples are Forensic teams for offender patients, Rehabilitation teams for individuals with high levels of enduring disabilities, Drug and Alcohol teams and Learning Disability teams. All of these have highly variable configurations. New personality disorder teams are soon to be established nationally in the UK on a local, though not catchment area, basis.

A third group comprises 'super-specialized' teams. These are not evenly spread and do not really aim to be comprehensive. Teams such as eating disorder teams or PTSD teams or those for the pre-lingually deaf often operate at a National or Regional level and take referrals from local services. They are essentially institution based (the patients travel to them) although they do often share much of the working practices which characterize CMHTs and other highly specialized teams.

Age specific teams

Old-age services

The profile of mental health problems changes with age. Paranoid and depressive disorders become more common and dementia poses probably the heaviest burden. The general health of older people deteriorates so that presentations to psychiatrists are often complicated (or may even be caused) both by physical illnesses and by the treatments of those illnesses. Old-age psychiatrists have to be much more alert, for example, to the possibilities of confusion or depression resulting from electrolyte imbalance or anaemia, or from the iatrogenic effects of polypharmacy for physical disorders, than is common in younger patients. The impact of increasing cognitive impairment and that of increasing physical frailty colour the work of old-age teams.

Domiciliary assessment and care

Home based assessments and domicilliary practice have been routine in old-age teams for decades – the '*in-vivo*' approach of ACT teams is nothing new to them. This was driven by the need to assess accurately cognitive impairment and day-to-day functioning. Mildly demented patients often appear very disabled and confused when in strange settings such as an outpatient department. It can be a remarkable surprise when they are seen at home where they are familiar with their surroundings and have highly evolved routines for conducting their lives. Proper risk assessment of a frail, dementing individual requires as much attention to the environment (e.g. steep stairs, open fires etc.) as to mental state. Travelling to appointments can also be difficult for patients with limited mobility.

Multidisciplinary practice

Multidisciplinary working has tended to be less fraught in old-age teams than with their general adult counterparts. There is less role blurring as the specific social, medical, and nursing needs are often clearer in the elderly. Roles could be seen as slightly more 'traditional' for this reason – nurses giving direct personal care, both physical and emotional, social workers organizing respite care and family support, and psychologists managing behavioural assessments and interventions. Because of the intimate interplay between physical and mental health in this age group, psychiatrists generally seem more established in their medical identities. Psychotherapies of differing sorts are currently receiving considerable attention in older patients.

Age of transition

Internationally, and even within the UK, there is variation in the age of transition for old-age teams. In the UK it is consolidating at 65 years although it was 70 or 75 years in some of the earlier teams. As the age cut-off lowers the balance between generic mental health care and a more purely dementia service alters. Some of the earlier services were focused exclusively on cognitive impairment, some even defined themselves as 'dementia only' services. The current emphasis in the Anglophone world is towards a more generic approach (in some European settings dementia is the responsibility of geriatricians, not psychiatrists at all).

The establishment of specific services for older patients has generally been considered a resounding success. The benefits are obvious in terms of increased expertise in managing frail and cognitively impaired individuals, and in terms of an enhanced commitment to comprehensive assessment and care across their multiple health and social care needs. Additionally it has ring-fenced resources and manpower for a previously very neglected group – and one that traditionally does not complain. Remarkably a charge of 'ageism' has been laid at this approach and currently there are moves to blur the concept of an age cut-off and emphasize individual needs assessment for access to different services. There are good arguments on both sides of this debate. It will be interesting to see how this evolves both in old-age services and in Child and Adolescent services where the same arguments are being rehearsed.

Child and adolescent services

Child and Adolescent Mental Health Services (CAMHS) have undergone massive changes in the last few decades. Thirty years ago most CAMHS teams were devoted to detailed and protracted assessments of children and families. Teams were multidisciplinary but with sharply delineated roles. CAMHS was probably the last bastion of the old practice of the psychiatrist assessing the patient and the social worker simultaneously meeting separately with the family and the two then meeting to decide what was to be done. Psychologists and psychotherapists on the teams had very clearly defined skills and roles, and usually only became involved with patients or families after they had been exhaustively assessed by the psychiatrists and social workers. They had very small caseloads and saw their patients for extended and extensive treatments. Some of the most sophisticated 'case work' practice was to be found by CAMHS social workers. Not surprisingly turnover was slow and waiting lists enormous. The standing joke among GPs was that half of the patients referred had grown out of the problem before they got an assessment.

An era of change

This sheltered 'provider driven' approach is long gone. CAMHS teams are now at the forefront of high-risk child protection cases and controversial issues such as those around attention deficit disorders. As a result team functioning has moved from the caricature above to a robust and flexible format closer to the adult CMHT. The disciplinary spread is broadly similar to adult CMHTs although there is often a higher prominence for psychologists who manage programmes for behavioural difficulties and social workers carry a very heavy responsibility in child protection cases. Multi-agency working with police, education, and social services forms a significant part of practice.

Like generic adult CMHTs, CAMHS teams have to provide prompt assessments for very undifferentiated problems. Identifying mental illnesses from within the range of adult distress and disorganization presenting at their surgery is difficult enough for GPs – how much more difficult having to make allowances for differing levels of maturity and development. Most teams allow for initial assessments by the full range of professionals with a significant triage function.

Inpatient provision

Inpatient provision is a much smaller component of CAMH services. If young people do need to be admitted then they almost invariably transfer to the care of a dedicated inpatient team. There are major problems with admissions for adolescents. Because youth inpatient services are few and far between there may be no local bed available for an acute psychotic episode (often the first breakdown) in a teenager. It is a counsel of perfection that they should be admitted to a dedicated age-appropriate ward (see Chapter 5). This may not be possible and often they are admitted to adult wards, especially if they are over 16 years of age. The maturity of 16–18 year olds can vary enormously. Some are still obviously terrified children while others are large, fully-grown, and insisting on their independence. Individualized sensitive decisions are needed which balance urgency against optimal care and specialism against the benefits of staying near to family and friends.

Age of transition

CAMH services have now moved their upper age of responsibility from 16 to 18 years. In some services youngsters between the ages of 16 and 18 were routed to CAMH or Adult services dependent on whether or not they were in full time education but this is increasingly seen as an unhelpful distinction. More recently there has been a move to blur age ranges in targeting CAMH services. The argument is that it is *developmental* rather than *chronological* age that matters. This makes sense where a CAMH service keeps on working with a patient who is over 18 but whose problems are still rooted in developmental or family issues. It makes very little sense in acute work or in disputed cases where clarity of *responsibility* is the vital issue. Here a simple age-based agreement about responsibility with the exercise of sensible clinical flexibility in management would seem the safest.

Disputes around age cut-offs have generally centred on the care of severely mentally ill young people. The problems have been most acute in settings where CAMH services have held more to the outdated model outlined above, and in particular where some senior psychiatrists had abrogated their responsibilities for managing such ill patients. There are still occasional (though increasingly rare) cases of Child psychiatrists asking their adult colleagues to prescribe Lithium for 16-year-old bipolar patients because they 'no longer feel competent to do so'. In Australia this has been the focus of considerable debate. Adult psychiatrists were seen as having successfully accepted an 'evidence based practice' approach to their work with CAMHS colleagues lagging, wedded more to a 'psychotherapy' approach. This was one strand in the Australian decision to move towards a 'youth service' (see Chapter 5) where adolescent care is absorbed more into adult team practice.

Teams serving special populations

Most well-developed local services have specialized teams serving adult patients whose mental health problems are complicated by specific, but fairly common complications. Forensic psychiatry teams provide care for mentally disordered offenders – where mental illnesses have involved criminal behaviour or are associated with significant levels of danger or threat. They may also have a specific remit for individuals with personality disorders or sexual behaviours who pose substantial risks.

Drug and alcohol misuse are widespread in mental health populations (as in the general population). Teams to help individuals with substance abuse and addictions are well established in most areas. There is an enormous variation in how they are organized and whether or not they will deal with people who are co-morbid for both substance abuse and mental illness.

Whether rehabilitation services are provided by a separate team or from within generic CMHTs and AO teams also varies from location to location. Well-developed rehabilitation teams are generally found either in metropolitan settings or in areas close to where large mental hospitals have closed and where they have reprovided for their long-stay population.

Learning disability services have experienced major upheavals in the last 30 years. Clarifying the role of the mental health professional in the overall social and personal care of individuals with learning disabilities has been highly controversial. In many settings the lead has been taken by social services leaving only a very limited role for the mental health team, others display highly developed, integrated working.

Forensic mental health teams

All forensic services serve courts and give advice to prisons and many have developed expertise in helping victims of crime. In many areas forensic services do this and provide medium secure care for mentally disordered offenders who pose serious risks and require quite protracted inpatient care. Some forensic psychiatrists insist that this is the correct extent of their services and that patients well enough to survive outside hospital should be freed of their forensic label.

Integrated and parallel services

The above is usually referred to as an '*integrated*' approach – care is integrated with generic or rehabilitation services. There is merit in this argument, especially applied to patients whose offending behaviour is limited to periods when they are unwell (e.g. those with psychoses). It is less appropriate in the context of patients who come to forensic services because of personality or sexual problems. Few general psychiatrists are well versed in the assessment of risk posed by sexual offenders. For such patients continuity of care with follow up is clearly indicated. Comprehensive long-term forensic services (both inpatient and outpatient) are called a '*parallel*' approach. They mirror the range of services provided by generic CMHTs but for their specialized patient population.

Expansion of forensic psychiatry

The last 10 years has seen forensic psychiatry extend its activity beyond the courtroom and secure hospital (Burns 2001; Snowden 2002). The usual model reflects generic CMHT structure and practice, although caseloads are smaller and some forensic services have set up assertive outreach teams. Forensic teams tend to work with their patients for several years and do not have a significant volume of short-term acute work. This more predictable work pattern promotes clearer role differentiation within these teams (as it does in diagnosis-specific services). The most obvious differences characterizing these teams is the increased attention they have to pay to risk assessment and their involvement in some of the complex legal provisions attached to their patients.

Drugs and alcohol teams

Drug and alcohol teams take a variety of forms. In some the services for drug abusers are separate from those for alcohol users, in some they are combined. Some services target patients with co-morbid severe mental health problems and some exclude them from their services; some take emergencies and some insist on high motivation and self-referral; still others are located in general hospitals and target early substance abuse. It is a clinical area rife with variation (including some settings where integration with general adult mental health teams is being tried). It is hardly possible to describe a typical team.

Harm-minimization and social stabilization

Drug and alcohol services generally emphasize a non-medical and non-judgemental approach. Increasingly harm-minimization approaches (e.g. needle exchanges) have come to be as important as treatments to address the addiction (e.g. detoxification, motivational interviewing). The approach is generally long-term with a focus on social stabilization and inclusion. The ethos of such teams is often explicitly casual – their clientele are generally uncomfortable with authority figures, so suits and professional titles are fairly scarce.

As with psychosis-care, relapses are a routine part of the job and expectations must be realistic. Even more than their general psychiatry counterparts drug and alcohol teams work in a highly politicized environment at the interface between health care and the criminal justice system. In the UK, for instance, significant funding streams may stem from the government departments primarily responsible for police and prisons.

Rehabilitation teams

Rehabilitation teams target patients characterized more by enduring disabilities than episodic bouts of illness. Obviously this is a fairly subjective judgement, not a simple yes–no observation. Differences in functioning in patients between relapse and remission are infinitely variable. Some patients (e.g. some bipolar patients) recover fully and dramatically despite very severe episodes whereas with others (e.g. delusional disorders and schizophrenia) it may be more a matter of gradual shifts in level of functioning.

Deinstitutionalization and resettlement

In the 1970s and 1980s rehabilitation teams expanded as the deinstitution movement gained momentum. They settled the majority of long-stay patients outside hospitals in domestic scale accommodation with varying degrees of supervision and support. Most rehabilitation teams adopted a generic CMHT approach but with a significantly greater proportion of their work being predictable and routine. Emergencies do occur but social and psychological support on a day-to-day basis are the necessity for this very disabled patient group. An emphasis on occupation and leisure is prominent in rehabilitation teams – it is not enough to get patients well but to make sure that their lives have the potential for being rewarding. Reducing stigma and encouraging social inclusion are essential components of this. For example, one rehabilitation team became actively involved in educating local inhabitants about the needs of the residents of one of their supported houses and invited them in to dispel preconceptions (Wolff et al. 1996a, b).

Old and new long-stay patients

As the resettlement initiative has now essentially finished with the closure of the large mental hospitals the role of rehabilitation teams (how they differ from general adult services) has become less clear. Where general adult CMHTs concentrate on the severe and enduringly mentally ill (as they increasingly do in urban settings) then they will also spend a considerable part of their time caring for long-term disabled individuals, many of whom are supported in supervised accommodation. Much of their work would previously have been considered 'rehabilitation'. From the other direction the mix of old long-stay and new long-stay patients (Hirsch et al. 1979) in rehabilitation services is shifting the focus of their work to more unstable patients, often complicated by substance abuse and behavioural disturbances. There is an inevitable coming together of the two approaches.

A separate service or an integrated function?

Whether or not a separate rehabilitation service is needed is probably more a matter of local morbidity levels and treatment cultures, rather than a deeply ideological issue (though often presented as such). There are cogent arguments on both sides – the usual ones that have surfaced several times in this book around the balance between the values of skill development and those of generic working. This conceptual debate is played out vividly in local decisions about which directorate assertive outreach teams are located in – rehabilitation or general adult. There are no obvious major differences in the patient population served, nor indeed in the approach to the work, yet one team insists that it is a 'rehabilitation continuing care team' and the other that it is an 'intensive acute team' focusing on enduring disorders.

Learning disability teams

For a long period psychiatrists took a leading role in the care of individuals with learning disabilities although their needs were predominantly social and educational. The last 30 years has, quite rightly, seen this challenged with a distinction of the social care and support from the need for psychiatric input. The latter has increasingly been reserved for those individuals with learning disabilities who also have concurrent mental illnesses or behavioural disorders. In many areas this change was associated with an exaggerated political rhetoric. The contribution of the psychiatrist was not so much refined and focused, as attacked and denied. Subsequently several services found themselves in crisis because they had stripped out their mental health expertise and had to rely on general psychiatrists who were unfamiliar with the needs of their clients. This pendulum seems to be swinging back to a recognition of the limited, but vital, role that specialized mental health services have for those with both learning disabilities and mental illnesses.

Models of community care in this population closely parallel those in rehabilitation and general adult services although there is more inter-agency work and often much more opportunity to work with families. The psychotherapeutic needs of this group have lately been recognized and several teams are engaged in imaginative and innovative work.

Super-specialized teams

'Super-specialized' teams exist to provide care for rare problems which cannot be economically provided for within each local health care system. Few of them have a community component – their regional or national remit means that they are rarely able to provide outreach. Patients travel to them, usually for inpatient care or follow up in outpatient clinics.

Such services are usually multidisciplinary in form although with a highly variable range of professions. Patients are referred to them because of what they do – they do not have to adapt significantly to different patient needs. So, for example, a team established to treat chronic fatigue disorder using CBT will be mainly comprised of psychologists trained in the approach and leave social and overall medical care to the referring team. An eating disorder team may have psychotherapists (with either a nursing or psychology background) and dieticians predominating. There is very little role-blurring at all in these highly specialized teams and usually no emergency or duty provision.

Super-specialist teams have usually arisen around the special interest of individual senior clinicians. Not surprisingly they tend to be idiosyncratic and little would be achieved describing them here in detail. The current plan in the UK to establish a national coverage of teams for the care of people with personality disorder in a consistent manner will repay careful observation. Charismatic and talented individuals have driven the few examples that do exist. Will replicating the format replicate the outcomes? A trial of just such a replication is currently under way to test its feasibility in Democratic Therapeutic Communities based on the Henderson Hospital.

Conclusions

The basic principles and practice of multidisciplinary working which were developed in generic CMHTs have informed most other teams. This includes these specialized ones although there are some fairly consistent differences in emphasis. There is generally less role blurring in specialized teams. Clarity of roles becomes increasingly established the more specific the team's remit (the more 'homogenous' the patient group treated). Being able to predict and plan for anticipated needs means that roles can be more explicit. In particular the reduced input to urgent work and screening a wide range of possible problems means that the balance between assessment and treatment is shifted. Skills are refined, but flexibility is abandoned.

The establishment of specialized teams, even if their work practices are very similar (e.g. old-age psychiatry) has the important advantage of ring-fencing resources for patient groups which are easily overlooked or neglected. Most of the teams described in this chapter command broad clinical support for their necessity. It is important to recognize, however, that professionals invariably tend to stress the uniqueness of their skills and the difference between what they do from what their colleagues do. This drive to increasing specialization can be the source of valuable innovation and lead to improved care. It is also often driven by 'Empire Building'. The benefits of specialization are usually obvious. The costs, however, may be considerable but less acknowledged. It behoves service planners to weigh the balance carefully to avoid waste and inefficiency.

CHAPTER 8

The wider context and the research and development agenda

The move from large mental hospitals as the cornerstone of care to local and community based services is an international phenomenon. It is all too easy to view it as a discrete historical episode with a beginning and an end, starting from one event, or from one centre, with its effects diffusing across time and geography. Organizing the untidy and variable changes that have characterized this movement into some form of narrative helps make sense of it (for simplicity one must start somewhere). There is, however, a risk in this of producing a '*March of Progress*' caricature of reality. Just as there was no discrete and obvious start there is no obvious goal or final conclusion. It would be probably better to see the changes described in this book (whether they be historical, or the different team structures described) more as aspects of the continuous change that are part and parcel of all mental health services.

The importance of wider social developments

Wider social changes have often been directly responsible for changes in mental health care (e.g. the increased emphasis on personal liberties and rights after World War II, see Chapter 1). Even where a social change is not the direct cause of developments in mental health thinking (not a *sufficient* condition) it may provide an appropriate environment for them to take effect (a *necessary* condition).

Climate of opinion

Social changes can make new ideas (or even old, rejected ideas) relevant and acceptable. For example the post-war climate of a more inclusive society with a commitment to greater equality made the previously known, grim conditions of mental hospitals quite unacceptable.

Practical provisions

Social changes may also provide the necessary structures which are essential for new mental health thinking to be feasible. The egalitarian ethos of social inclusion of the late 1940s and 1950s could not have resulted in deinstitutionalization if the Welfare State had not been established. It was this welfare state that secured the financial and health care support outside institutions for these disabled individuals unable to work, and without families to care for them.

International variation

The differences between health care cultures from ostensibly similar countries may have profound impacts on the effectiveness of a particular service approach. Well-established primary care, or the successful integration of health and social care will undoubtedly influence the relative effectiveness of a mental health team in discharging its tasks. Indeed they will also probably subtly affect the very tasks the team views as its responsibility. Yet these contextual factors have very rarely been commented on in the research literature, or recognized as essential considerations in transferring mental health service research from one country to another (Burns 2000*b*). This neglect is even more remarkable when Mangen (Mangen 1985) reported that even such an epoch-making event as the introduction of chlorpromazine in the 1950s had substantially different impacts in different European countries.

International developments

Anglophone cultures (the UK, USA, and Australia) have been very prominent in mental health services research. This reflects a strongly established scientific culture and (in Australia and the UK) of centrally organized and funded services. There is also a language bias in academic publications where English dominates. There has been no shortage, however, of innovation and excellence internationally. Most of the basic principles and practices of CMHTs, as described in the preceding chapters, are found in these different cultures. The priorities and emphases, however, vary to reflect local differences and attitudes.

Change is also rapid in most European countries as deinstitutionalization has driven the community care agenda (albeit at different rates). Familiarity with writings from some of these different approaches to mental health care can teach us much and improve our ability to plan and develop better services for the future. Probably almost every country in the world has something interesting to contribute to better planning and delivery of community mental health. It is not, however, feasible to do justice to them all in a book like this. The main cultural variations that shape the history and current developments have been selected for mention. This is a very rough and ready selection – based on experience of what gets quoted and compared. It is inevitably partial and incomplete.

The Italian Revolution, 'Law 180'

Probably the most dramatic upheaval in recent community mental health practice was that which occurred in Italy at the end of the 1970s. Led by a charismatic and politically astute psychiatrist Franco Bassaglia the 'Psichiatria Democratica' movement was launched (Mangen 1989). Bassaglia was a well trained and forward thinking social psychiatrist who had travelled and studied abroad as well as in his native Italy. He returned to take up a senior position, eventually in Trieste where he initiated his reforms. Conditions in the mental hospital were truly awful. Bassaglia brought not just a reforming psychiatrist's perspective to the task but also that of a Gramsian Marxist. He emphasized the power relationships within psychiatry as *the* major problem and set about a structural change with freedom and equality (rather than simply improved care) as the primary goals. This manifested itself in the famous 'Law 180' in 1978 (Mangen 1989).

Hospital reforms

Under this new law admissions to mental hospitals were prohibited and inpatient care was transferred to the new 'diagnostic units' – 15 bedded wards in acute hospitals. Compulsory treatment was restricted to patients posing a risk of harm and limited to a maximum of a week (although this could be renewed repeatedly). ECT was effectively banned from public mental health care. Mental hospitals were given 3 years to reprovide for their patients. In practice the radical reforms were implemented well in the North of Italy but not consistently throughout the country (Fioritti *et al.* 1997) and attracted both admiration and criticism in abundance (Jones and Poletti 1985).

Community practice

The CMHTs that arose in response to the Italian reforms have a special flavour. They are generally very positive and self-confident with an emphasis on generalism. In Italy there has not been the development of the specialized teams that have dominated elsewhere. Italian university departments tend to deal with the specialist populations and the public sector services with community psychiatry. Also, given the extensive network of private and insurance based services, Italian CMHTs have an exclusive focus on the SMI. They usually comprise the CMHT and the inpatient ward as a single team and demonstrate more flexibility of work between the two areas than do UK or US services. Thus home follow up of a patient recently discharged may very likely be by the 'inpatient' nurse who has worked with them during the admission. Transfer between inpatient and day care is informal and easy. Day patients come to the resource centre or the ward depending on local arrangements. Food, not surprisingly for Italy, is an important part of care and cooked on site and a significant attraction for attendance.

The language of Italian CMHTs is up-beat and empowering. The informality of relationships between staff and patients is striking. Contrary to what many visitors expect, however, treatment is firmly based on medication and routines (Italian psychiatrists prescribe significantly more psychotropics than their UK counterparts). Like other Mediterranean services they can rely on the family for social care much more than in northern Europe or the US. Doctors have generally been plentiful in Italy (there is currently substantial medical unemployment) so there has not been the same drive for other disciplines to share responsibility (Burns *et al.* 2001).

The French 'Secteur'

France was very active in the 1960s and 1970s in its development of community mental health services. The French *secteur* had quite different intellectual origins but ended up remarkably similar to the early UK sector. They were organized around hospital catchment areas and geographical team sectors (Kovess *et al.* 1995). Traditionally French psychiatrists have been more concerned with having a coherent theoretical base for their practice as compared to the more pragmatic UK. The *secteur* arose more from sociological considerations of care provision than the practicalities of co-ordinating teams.

Crisis centres were also established in hospital casualty departments where particular attention has been paid to suicide prevention. This is not surprising in one of the birthplaces of modern sociology where Durkheim's groundbreaking study was published (Durkheim 1897). In recent decades, however, French psychiatry has been somewhat uncommunicative with international practice. Psychoanalysis still has a prominent position (even in the public sector) and the complexities of the particularly impenetrable French brand of psychoanalysis fostered by Lacan (Lacan 1966) have entrenched this isolation. The high regard for psychoanalysis, however, ensures careful attention to the human and interpersonal aspects of mental health care and visitors return impressed by services. Obtaining a coherent overview of current community services is, however, difficult.

Northern European influences

Inpatient: community divide

Scandinavia and the German-speaking countries have their own traditions of community mental health care. The most striking differences to the UK (apart from the obvious high level of investment) is that there is often a separation between inpatient care and community care – the very opposite of the Italian approach. In Germany there were, until recently, legal barriers in most provinces against continuity of care across the hospital – outpatient divide. These rules were to prevent restrictive practices (care is predominantly insurance based, fee for service). There is still, as in many parts of the US, a large body of private practitioners working purely in outpatients. Several German provinces have moved away from this to develop continuity of care, usually based on a case-management system.

German social psychiatry

In Germany social psychiatry has a more 'radical' connotation than it does elsewhere. In the past it has, indeed, overlapped with 'anti-psychiatry'. Social workers have been the dominant discipline and usually worked as the case managers for the severely mentally ill. Some German commentators have characterized the case-management and ACT movements simply as a rebadging exercise with Health Care claiming credit for well-established social work practices.

In Scandinavia and the Netherlands the same hospital/community split is still common. However, the professional inputs to the teams is much more like that described in the UK with a mixture of nurses, social workers, occupational therapists, and clinical psychologists. Scandinavian countries and the Netherlands have been much more open to international trends such as the development of Assertive Outreach teams and Early Intervention teams.

North America

Any visitor to the USA quickly learns not to generalize. Services in different states differ as much between them as they do between European countries. Some states have highly developed and comprehensive care for the severely mentally ill, others provide little beyond emergency and inpatient care for those who pose a serious risk to those around them. Deinstitutionalization started later but progressed faster than in the UK with predicable consequences (Chapter 1). The US has been a hotbed of innovation as centres of excellence have risen to the challenge of displaced severely disabled individuals. Case-management was the first response (Intagliata 1982), and ACT (Stein and Test 1980) its most influential development.

The absence of a comprehensive approach to mental health care in the US is a severe problem for patients and their families. However, it has meant that innovators have been free to specialize and experiment in ways that would be almost unthinkable in most of Europe. The US team is defined by the clinical characteristics of its target patients. Their ability to exclude patients who do not fully meet their remit means that they can refine their practices to very high standards, e.g. specific services for dual diagnosis patients (Drake *et al.* 1995), or for homeless patients (Drake *et al.* 1997). Not surprisingly US demonstration services serve as laboratories of innovation and excellence. While this undoubtedly helps move the agenda forward it can, sometimes, be at the cost of careful reflection and attention to context and variance.

Australia

Australian psychiatrists (Edwards *et al.* 2000; Hoult *et al.* 1984) have been very prominent in promoting service developments in community psychiatry. In particular they have taken the ACT and EIS approaches forward and become international champions for them. Their mid-position reflects a European commitment to comprehensive care (and hence the inertia that goes with it) with a more vigorous American 'can-do' approach. The UK has certainly benefited from their close links.

The wider international scene

The focus on European and Anglophone services and research in this brief overview does not mean there are not excellent services and innovations elsewhere. There are – although we should not delude ourselves about the very poor standards of care for most patients across the globe. In particular some of the developing countries have evolved cost-effective approaches to mental health, which are based on community resources and a *public health* approach. Many have neither the resources nor the desire to replicate the asylum building phase from 19th century Europe and America. They are not addressed here because to do so would have to be inevitably ramdom, and also because interpreting their relevance would be a mammoth task, well beyond the remit of this book.

The importance of 'unimportant' activity

Not all change is innovation

Innovation is not enough. To be a worthwhile innovation (not simply a 'change') a service development must demonstrate that it produces better outcomes than that which precedes it. Not only that, it must be sustainable (Coid 1994). What makes services successful and what makes them sustainable and generalizable is often not clear at the outset. Contrast the impact of the original highly successful ACT study (Stein and Test 1980) and an equally successful acute day hospital study (Creed *et al.* 1990). Why does one conquer the world and one remain barely replicated?

Professional identity and needs

Ostensibly unimportant details may sometimes be critical in sustaining the success of a service development. An example of this is found in the dispersal of community mental health teams. In the 1970s and early 1980s there was a move to locate CMHTs away from the hospital to emphasize their 'communitiness' and improve access. For financial and practical reasons this could not always be achieved. Theoretically a stand alone CMHT in an inconspicuous converted house in a road should provide a better service (more accessible, less stigmatizing, less medical model). In reality these dispersed services soon developed more than their fair share of problems. They have generally survived less well than apparently more compromised services that had to use more institutional premises.

It has become clear that, after the initial enthusiasm, staff generally find working in such isolated settings difficult. The professional structures that were thought (probably correctly) to stand in the way of a more holistic approach were revealed as having other less obvious benefits such as maintaining confidence and job satisfaction. Their importance goes beyond there being a canteen or some duty-cover. Regular contact with other professionals also ensured that standards do not drift and a sense of proportion is maintained. In truth the role played by a clear professional identity in withstanding the stresses and strains of mental health work only became clear when it was removed.

Sustaining a service

The same holds for many of the aspects of running a service that often seem 'secondary' or unimportant but prove to be vital to ensure their continued well-being. Virtually anything is possible for a few years if people are sufficiently enthused and motivated. Staff may work excessive hours or impossible rotas, or contain absurdly high levels of stress and uncertainty as part of the 'buzz' of a new service. To sustain a service, however, it needs both to meet patients' needs and also the staff's legitimate needs – effective for the patient but also professionally rewarding. Staff also need adequate administrative support and professional development – there must be ongoing training and a meaningful career structure with the possibility of promotion. It can be very tempting to put all resources into front-line clinical input and neglect management and support functions, but this soon begins to tell.

Relationships with colleagues

Relationships with surrounding services need to be honest and respectful. Some very innovative services have neglected relationships with those around them, sometimes making their colleagues feel 'old hat' or even looked down upon. They have been surprised when those colleagues have not backed them up or supported them when they subsequently needed it. Really enthused and radical services often dismiss the energies and time devoted to professional matters as stuffy or irrelevant. Experience teaches otherwise.

Adapting to the environment

Darwinian evolutionists have taught us that the fundamental measure of success is whether a species (here *service*) survives and flourishes. This requires us to make more inclusive judgements. We do our patients no favours if we deliver a 20% improvement in care from a wonderful but unsustainable service which results, 5 years on, in a collapse leaving no provision at all.

Both day hospitals and inpatients units have experienced a major change in their functioning in the last 30 years because of the increasing capacity of CMHTs and other community teams to deal with more seriously ill patients in their own homes. As a result inpatient wards and day hospitals running sophisticated milieu therapy programmes foundered. The nature of patients admitted had changed so dramatically that their previously successful approach was successful no longer. The change in the clinical challenge did not reflect a change in the prevalence or severity of disorders but more a change in the behaviour of another player in the system (i.e. the CMHT).

Attention to context

It will be obvious from the tone of this book that it is failure to acknowledge the impact of the inter-relations of different services that causes misunderstanding and dispute. All too often the success of an approach is presented as if it lay entirely within its internal structure. There is inadequate attention to its relationships to services that support and work with it or, more crucially, the services with which it is compared.

No research study of a mental health service is conducted against a placebo. Service studies are always comparisons between at least two services (even if one is very underdeveloped, it is still *a service*). The 'success' demonstrated by a research study for any proposed configuration is its advantage over its competitor. It is not inherent – despite current preoccupations with model fidelity.

The research agenda

Research and evaluation are accepted responsibilities of competent health service providers. We live in an increasingly 'Evidence Based' culture and few would doubt the overall value of this development. Despite the occasional criticisms that it can lead to lack of originality or sensitivity to the unique individual patient (Clinicians for the Restoration of Autonomous Practice (CRAP) Writing Group 2002) it protects patients and practitioners alike.

The evidence base for different CMHT practices can only be obtained by collaboration of such teams with the research agenda. This is often an unwelcome extra burden on top of clinical audit and local demands for evaluation. Research is different from audit and evaluation.

Clinical audit and service evaluation

Audit is testing current practice against known and accepted standards. It does not tell us anything new about how to practice but how we compare with the practice of others. Evaluations are an increasing feature of modern practice. As service innovations represent a redeployment of clinical resources from one system (the 'old model of care') into another (the 'new model of care') the question is asked 'are we getting equal, or better value from the new service?' This 'value' is usually measured in health benefit for patients or, more often, the use of inpatient care (generally viewed as excessively expensive and to be avoided where possible). New services are almost invariably more expensive than those they replace (initiating a new service is increasingly the only way to obtain increased investment). Thus the evaluation is expected to demonstrate an improvement in outcome – either less reliance on beds, reduced waiting times, or some broad measure of satisfaction or quality of life.

Limited generalizability of evaluations

Service evaluations are not conducted with the rigor that characterizes research proper. The main limitations of service evaluations are that they can only indicate whether *this innovation* is superior or not to its predecessor *in this location*. It does not tell you whether the approach is superior overall; its results are not generalizable. If I show that my new day hospital reduces inpatient admissions compared to the old one it does not necessarily mean that *your* new day hospital will. Your day hospital may be very different from mine.

Research, however, seeks to maximize the generalizability of its findings. All the complex and detailed procedures that characterize careful research (sample selection, manualization of programmes, randomization, blinding of raters etc.) are to minimize bias and increase generalizability. Even when all these precautions have been taken the generalizability of any one study is still limited. Most researchers would acknowledge that they cannot guarantee total generalizability – what they aim to achieve is that the degree and limits of the generalizability can be fairly confidently known. A research study should be described in sufficient detail that it is accurately repeatable.

Research into complex interventions

The burgeoning of different forms of CMHT appears to offer almost limitless research opportunities. Many new teams want to 'do a study' comparing their performance, usually against the situation before their development or using their neighbour as the comparator. This is how the first generation of community mental health studies were conducted. If the results were positive they encouraged further development and research. If not, then it was time to think again.

Research into complex systems such as mental health teams is now, however, well beyond this simple paradigm. It remains, however, the first step in evaluating a novel approach – testing its overall performance against routine care (usually now called 'Treatment as Usual', TAU). A more sharply focused design with carefully worded hypotheses and careful choice of outcome measures is now needed for any real assessment of the benefits and drawbacks of new teams or new variations.

Limitations of head-to-head trials

Simple head-to-head trials tell us increasingly little. We need to ensure we know which of the several components of the complex intervention differ between the two arms of a trial (whether randomized or case controlled). We need to control carefully for bias in the context (is the supporting environment the same for both conditions?), and in the staffing and training across the services. It has become increasingly important to be very explicit about defining the outcome to be measured and to do this *before* conducting the study. Too often research studies have measured a wide range of outcomes and then simply reported those that showed differences, ignoring those that did not.

In dealing with variable, relapsing-remitting disorders such as the major psychoses it can be possible to affect outcomes such as satisfaction with services, quality of life etc., while still not showing significant differences in symptom levels and vice versa. The choice of outcome is both crucial and difficult. One needs to know considerable details about the likely distribution of the chosen measure to work out how large the study must be to 'prove' a difference.

In short, mental health services research with complex interventions such as those delivered by CMHTs is not for the faint-hearted or busy. To be meaningful the studies need to be very carefully thought through, rigorously conducted and realistic in their expectations. As much time needs to be spent thinking through the questions to be addressed as in carrying out the study. Is the question clinically or theoretically important? Can it be convincingly answered by the chosen study design? Can bias and confounding be successfully reduced or, at least, accounted for? How generalizable is the intervention and the answer?

The future research agenda

The UK government, through the medium of the National Institute for Mental Health for England (NIMHE), is actively evolving a strategy for mental health research to raise quality, avoid redundancy and duplication, and ensure that clinically important areas are addressed. The emphasis is on promoting collaborative work with multisite studies (essential to get sufficient 'power' to answer questions convincingly, and also to avoid the bias introduced by local champions) and on widening outcomes and methodologies. Traditional outcomes based on symptoms are being complemented by more 'user-generated' outcomes and those that relate to patients' and families' priorities, such as work, empowerment, and independence. Large, methodologically rigorous studies can be enhanced with qualitative work to capture the patient's experience of the process.

Development leads research – not vice versa

However, by its very nature the future research agenda cannot be accurately foreseen or planned. Nor can service development depend entirely on research for its progress. Research can only test whether or not a belief is correct – it does not generate the belief. Service developments come from theoretical (often from ideological) positions. The research tests whether the enthusiast's conviction that their innovation really is an improvement. Community psychiatry research is littered with excessive claims backed up by 'research' which has not been sufficiently sophisticated to answer the questions it has claimed to address (Coid 1994). What can be anticipated with some certainty is that the rigor of research in this field will increase. Questions will be more focused, controls tighter both within studies and at their margins. Statisticians and methodologists (both quantitative and qualitative) will be involved in the design of studies, not just in their analysis.

Conclusions

A review of Community Mental Health practice should probably not have a 'conclusions' section. The burden of this chapter has been to stress the inevitability of change and development within practice. It is not a case of 'a good idea' originating somewhere to solve 'the problem' and then various countries moving at different rates to implement that idea. Practice is always evolving, driven by both internal and external changes. Different countries and cultures throw up different challenges, perspectives and priorities. There are lots of different service configurations as there are also different ethical codes.

While cultural diversity has enriched community mental health teams, a more narrow nationalism has at times obstructed developments. Strong feelings, usually based on enthusiasm for a particular model, have often become polarized around national and regional 'camps'. This is not surprising but it is regrettable. An 'evolutionary' perspective would encourage a 'wait and see' approach about these developments. Time will tell which is better. Often this can be aided by high-quality research, but not always. Useful research will need to be increasingly sophisticated and careful if it is to make us any wiser – the era of simple, exciting, head-to-head trials is probably past.

The last 40 years have seen enormous changes in mental health care and the next 40 are likely to see even more. New understandings of the causes of the illnesses we treat will profoundly alter what CMHTs need to do and the training of those who do it. It is unlikely, however, that the multiprofessional approach that forms the bulk of this book will fade away. Unless some magic 'therapeutic bullet' is discovered the care of most of the severe mental illnesses will require collaboration and team work. The CMHT of 2040 may be very different from that of 2000 but it will probably remain recognizably a CMHT.

References

Allness, D. and Knoedler, W. (1998) *The PACT model of community based treatment for persons with severe and persistent mental illness: A manual for PACT start-up.* National Alliance for the Mentally Ill Anti-Stigma Campaign, Arlington VA.

American Psychiatric Association (1980) *Diagnostic and statistical manual of mental disorders* (3rd edn). American Psychiatric Association, Washington DC.

American Psychiatric Association (1994) *Diagnostic and statistical manual of mental disorders* (4th edn). American Psychiatric Association, Washington DC.

Amin, S., Singh, S. P., Croudace, T., Jones, P., Medley, I., and Harrison, G. (1999) Evaluating the Health of the Nation Outcome Scales. Reliability and validity in a three-year follow-up of first-onset psychosis. *British Journal of Psychiatry*, **174**, 399–403.

Anderson, J., Dayson, D., Wills, W., Gooch, C., Margolius, O., O'Driscoll, C., *et al.* (1993) The TAPS Project. 13: Clinical and social outcomes of long-stay psychiatric patients after one year in the community. *British Journal of Psychiatry – Supplement no.* **19**, 45–56.

Appleby, L., Shaw, J., Amos, T., McDonnell, R., Harris, C., McCann, K., *et al.* (1999) Suicide within 12 months of contact with mental health services: national clinical survey. *British Medical Journal*, **318**, 1235–9.

Arlidge, J. T. (1859) *On the state of lunacy and the legal provision for the insane, with observations on the construction and organization of asylums.* J&A Churchill, London.

Bachrach, L. L. (1988) Defining chronic mental illness: a concept paper. *Hospital & Community Psychiatry*, **39**(4), 383–8.

Bachrach, L. L. (1997) Lessons in the American experience in providing community-based services, in *Care in the Community: Illusion or Reality?* J. Leff, (ed.), John Wiley & Sons, Chichester.

Balint, M. (1968) *The doctor, his patient and the illness.* Pitman Medical, London.

Barnes, T. R. (1989) A rating scale for drug-induced akathisia. *British Journal of Psychiatry*, **154**, 672–6.

Barnes, T. R., Hutton, S. B., Chapman, M. J., Mutsatsa, S., Puri, B. K., and Joyce, E. M. (2000) West London first-episode study of schizophrenia: Clinical correlates of duration of untreated psychosis. *British Journal of Psychiatry*, **177**, 207–11.

Barton, R. (1959) *Institutional neurosis.* John Wright, Bristol.

Bateson, G., Jackson, D., Haley, J., and Weakland, J. (1956) Towards a theory of schizophrenia. *Behavioral Science*, **1**, 251–64.

Bauer, M., Kunze, H., Von Cranach, M., Fritze, J., and Becker, T. (2001) Psychiatric reform in Germany. *Acta Psychiatrica Scandinavica, Supplementum no.* **410**, 27–34.

Bebbington, P., Wilkins, S., Jones, P., Foerster, A., Murray, R., Toone, B., *et al.* (1993) Life events and psychosis. Initial results from the Camberwell Collaborative Psychosis Study. *British Journal of Psychiatry*, **162**, 72–9.

Beck, A. T., Ward, C. H., Mendelson, M., Mock, J. E., and Erbaugh, J. K. (1961) An inventory for measuring depression. *Archives of General Psychiatry*, **4**, 561–71.

Becker, D. R. and Drake, R. E. (1993) *A working life: The Individual Placement and Support (IPS) Program.* Dartmouth Psychiatric Research Center, New Hampshire.

Bell, G. M. (1955) A mental hospital with open doors. *International Journal of Social Psychiatry*, **1**, 42–8.

Bennett, D. (1991) The drive towards the community, in *150 Years of British Psychiatry 1841–1991.* G. E. Berrios and H. Freeman, (ed.), Gaskell, London, 321–32.

Bierer, J. (1951) *The Day Hospital* H&K Lewis, London.

Birchwood, M., Jackson, C., and Todd, P. (1998) The critical period hypothesis. *International Clinical Psychopharmacy*, **12**, 27–38.

Birchwood, M., McGorry, P., and Jackson, H. (1997) Early intervention in schizophrenia. *British Journal of Psychiatry*, **170**, 2–5.

Birchwood, M., Smith, J., MacMillan, F., Hogg, B., Prasad, R., Harvey, C., et al. (1989) Predicting relapse in schizophrenia: the development and implementation of an early signs monitoring system using patients and families as observers, a preliminary investigation. *Psychological Medicine*, **19**(3), 649–56.

Birchwood, M., Spencer, E., and McGovern, D. (2000) Schizophrenia: early warning signs. *Advances in Psychiatric Treatment*, **6**, 93–101.

Bisson, J. I., McFarlane, A. C., and Rose, S. (2000) Psychological debriefing, in *Effective treatments for PTSD: Practical guidelines from the International Society for Traumatic Stress Studies.* E. B. Foa, T. M. Keane, and M. J. Friedman, (ed.), Guildford Press, New York and London, 39–59.

Brewin, C. R., Wing, J. K., Mangen, S. P., Brugha, T. S., MacCarthy, B., and Lesage, A. (1988) Needs for care among the long-term mentally ill: a report from the Camberwell High Contact Survey. *Psychological Medicine*, **18**(2), 457–68.

Brill, H. and Patton, R. E. (1962) Clinical-statistical analysis of population changes in New York state mental hospitals since the introduction of psychotropic drugs. *American Journal of Psychiatry*, **119**, 20.

British Journal of Psychiatry (2000) HoNOS update. *British Journal of Psychiatry*, **176**, 392–5.

Brook, B. D. (1973) Crisis hostel: an alternative to psychiatric hospitalization for emergency patients. *Hospital & Community Psychiatry*, **24**(9), 621–4.

Brown, G. W., Birley, J. L., and Wing, J. K. (1972) Influence of family life on the course of schizophrenic disorders: a replication. *British Journal of Psychiatry*, **121**(562), 241–58.

Bucknill, J. C. (1858) Description of a new house at the Devon county lunatic asylum, with remarks upon the sea-side residence for the insane, which was for a time established at Exmouth. *Journal of Mental Science*, **4** , 317–28.

Burns, T. (2000*a*) Psychiatric home treatment. Vigorous, well designed trials are needed. *British Medical Journal*, **321**(7254), 177.

Burns, T. (2000*b*) Models of community treatments in schizophrenia: do they travel? *Acta Psychiatrica Scandinavica*, **102**(407), 11–14.

Burns, T. (2001) To outreach or not to outreach. *Journal of Forensic Psychiatry*, **12**(1), 13–17.

Burns, T. and Bale, R. (1997) Establishing a mental health liaison attachment with primary care. *Advances in Psychiatric Treatment*, **3**, 219–24.

Burns, T., Beadsmoore, A., Bhat, A. V., Oliver, A., and Mathers, C. (1993*a*) A controlled trial of home-based acute psychiatric services. I: Clinical and social outcome. *British Journal of Psychiatry*, **163**, 49–54.

Burns, T., Raftery, J., Beadsmoore, A., McGuigan, S., and Dickson, M. (1993*b*) A controlled trial of home-based acute psychiatric services. II: Treatment patterns and costs. *British Journal of Psychiatry*, **163**, 55–61.

Burns, T., Fiander, M., Kent, A., Ukoumunne, O. C., Byford, S., Fahy, T., *et al.* (2000) Effects of case load size on the process of care of patients with severe psychotic illness. *British Journal of Psychiatry*, **177**(427), 433.

Burns, T., Fioritti, A., Holloway, F., Malm, U., and Rossler, W. (2001) Case Management and Assertive Community Treatment in Europe. *Psychiatric Services*, **52**(5), 631–6.

Burns, T. and Firn, M. (2002*a*) *Assertive outreach in mental health: A manual for practitioners*. Oxford University Press, Oxford.

Burns, T. and Firn, M. (2002*b*) Key working versus the 'team approach', in *Assertive outreach in mental health: a manual for practitioners*. T. Burns and M. Firn, (ed.), Oxford University Press, Oxford.

Burns, T. and Firn, M. (2002*c*) Compulsion and freedom, in *Assertive outreach in mental health: a manual for practitioners*. T. Burns and M. Firn, (ed.), Oxford University Press, Oxford.

Burns, T. and Guest, L. (1999) Running an assertive community treatment team. *Advances in Psychiatric Treatment*, **5**, 348–56.

Burns, T. and Leibowitz, J. (1997) The Care Programme Approach: time for frank talking. *Psychiatric Bulletin*, **21**, 426–9.

Campbell, H., Hotchkiss, R., Bradshaw, N., and Porteous M. (1998) Critical care pathways. *British Medical Journal*, **316**, 133–7.

Caplan, G. (1961) *An approach to community mental health*. Grune and Stratton, New York.

Carse, J., Panton, N., and Watt, A. (1958) A district mental service: the Worthing experiment. *Lancet*, **i**, 39–41.

Castle, D. J. and Murray, R. M. (1993) The epidemiology of late-onset schizophrenia. *Schizophrenia Bulletin*, **19**(4), 691–700.

Catty, J. and Burns, T. (2001) Mental health day centres: Their clients and role. *Psychiatric Bulletin*, **25**, 61–6.

Catty, J., Burns, T., Knapp, M., Watt, H., Wright, C., Henderson, J., *et al.* (2002) Home treatment for mental health problems: A systematic review. *Psychological Medicine*, **32**, 383–401.

Chadwick, P. and Birchwood, M. (1994) The omnipotence of voices. A cognitive approach to auditory hallucinations. *British Journal of Psychiatry*, **164**(2), 190–201.

Chaplin, R., Gordon, J., and Burns, T. (1999) Early detection of antipsychotic side-effects. *Psychiatric Bulletin*, **23**, 657–60.

Chaplin, R. and Kent, A. (1998) Informing patients about tardive dyskinesia. Controlled trial of patient education. *British Journal of Psychiatry*, **172**, 78–81.

Child, J. (1977) *Organisation: A guide to problems and practice*. Harper and Row, New York.

Ciompi, L. (1988) Learning from outcome studies toward a comprehensive biological-psychosocial understanding of schizophrenia. *Schizophrenia Research*, **1**, 373–84.

Clement, S., Singh, S. P., and Burns, T. (2003) Status of bipolar disorder research: Bibliometric study. *British Journal of Psychiatry*, **182**, 148–52.

Clinicians for the Restoration of Autonomous Practice (CRAP) Writing Group (2002) EBM: unmasking the ugly truth. *British Medical Journal*, **325**(7378), 1496–8.

Coid, J. (1994) Failure in community care: psychiatry's dilemma. *British Medical Journal*, **308**(6932), 805–6.

Coid, J. W. (1996) Dangerous patients with mental illness: increased risks warrant new policies, adequate resources, and appropriate legislation. *British Medical Journal*, **312**(7036), 965–6.

Conolly, J. (1830) *An inquiry concerning the indications of insanity with suggestions for the better protection and care of the insane*. John Taylor, London.

Cooper, J. E. (1979) Crisis admission units and emergency psychiatric services. in *Public health in Europe*, No. 2, World Health Organization, Copenhagen.

Craig, T. J., Bromet, E. J., Fennig, S., Tanenberg-Karant, M., Lavelle, J., and Galambos, N. (2000) Is there an association between duration of untreated psychosis and 24-month clinical outcome in a first-admission series? *American Journal of Psychiatry*, **157**(1), 60–66.

Creed, F., Black, D., Anthony, P., Osborn, M., Thomas, P., and Tomenson, B. (1990) Randomised controlled trial of day patient versus inpatient psychiatric treatment. *British Medical Journal*, **300**(6731), 1033–7.

Davidson, J. R. (1997) Biological therapies for post traumatic stress disorder: an overview. *Journal of Clinical Psychiatry*, **58**(Suppl 9), 29–32.

Dayson, D. (1993) The TAPS Project. 12: Crime, vagrancy, death and readmission of the long-term mentally ill during their first year of local reprovision. *British Journal of Psychiatry – Supplement no.* **19**, 40–44.

de Girolamo, G., Picardi, A., Micciolo, R., Falloon, I., Fioritti, A., and Morosini, P. (2002) Residential care in Italy. National survey of non-hospital facilities. *British Journal of Psychiatry*, **181**, 220–5.

Deahl, M. and Turner, T. (1997) General psychiatry in no-man's land. *British Journal of Psychiatry*, **171**, 6–8.

Dean, C., Phillips, J., Gadd, E. M., Joseph, M., and England, S. (1993) Comparison of community based service with hospital based service for people with acute, severe psychiatric illness. *British Medical Journal*, **307**(6902), 473–6.

Department of Health (1990) *The Care Programme Approach for people with a mental illness referred to the Special Psychiatric Services*. Department of Health, London, Joint Health/Social Services Circular HC (90) 23/LASS (90) 11.

Department of Health (1999a) *Modern Standards and Service Models: National Service Framework for Mental Health*. Department of Health, London.

Department of Health (1999b) *Safer services: National Confidential Inquiry into suicide and homicide by people with mental illness*. Department of Health, London.

Department of Health (2000) *The NHS Plan – A plan for investment, a plan for reform*. Department of Health, London.

Department of Health (2001) *The Mental Health Policy Implementation Guide*. Department of Health, London.

Department of Health (2002) *Mental Health Policy Implementation Guide: Community Mental Health Teams*. Department of Health, London, 28165.

Department of Health and Social Security (1984) *Caring for people: Community care in the next decade and beyond, cmnd 849*. HMSO, London.

Department of Health and Social Services Inspectorate (1991) *Care management and assessment: Summary of practice guidelines*. HMSO, London.

Done, D. J., Crow, T. J., Johnstone, E. C., and Sacker, A. (1994) Childhood antecedents of schizophrenia and affective illness: social adjustment at ages 7 and 11. *British Medical Journal*, **309**(6956), 699–703.

Drake, R. E., Becker, D. R., Biesanz, J. C., Torrey, W. C., McHugo, G. J., and Wyzik, P. F. (1994) Rehabilitative day treatment vs. supported employment: I. Vocational outcomes. *Community Mental Health Journal*, **30**(5), 519–32.

Drake, R. E., McHugo, G. J., Bebout, R. R., Becker, D. R., Harris, M., Bond, G. R., et al. (1999) A randomized clinical trial of supported employment for inner-city patients with severe mental disorders. *Archives of General Psychiatry*, **56**(7), 627–33.

Drake, R. E., McHugo, G. J., Clark, R. E., Teague, G. B., Xie, H., Miles, K., et al. (1998) Assertive community treatment for patients with co-occurring severe mental illness and substance use disorder: A Clinical Trial. *American Journal of Orthopsychiatry*, **68**(2), 201–15.

Drake, R. E., Noordsy, D. L., and Ackerson, T. (1995) Integrating mental health and substance abuse treatments for persons with chronic mental disorders: A model, in *Double jeopardy: Chronic mental illness and substance abuse.* A. F. Lehman and L. B. Dixon, (ed.), Harwood Academic Publishers, Baltimore.

Drake, R. E., Yovetich, N. A., Bebout, R. R., Harris, M., and McHugo, G. J. (1997) Integrated treatment for dually diagnosed homeless adults. *Journal of Nervous & Mental Disease*, **185**(5), 298–305.

Durkheim, E. (1897) *Le Suicide: etude de sociologie.* Alcan, Paris.

Edwards, J., McGorry, P. D., and Pennell, K. (2000) Models of early intervention in psychosis: an analysis of service approaches, in *Early intervention in psychosis: a guide to concepts, evidence and interventions.* M. Birchwood, D. Fowler, and C. Jackson, (ed.), John Wiley & Sons, New York, 281–314.

Erikson, E. H. (1959) *Identity and the life cycle.* International Universities Press, New York.

Essex, B., Doig, R., and Renshaw, J. (1990) Pilot study of records of shared care for people with mental illnesses. *British Medical Journal*, **300**(6737), 1442–6.

Fenton, W. S. and McGlashan, T. H. (1994) Antecedents, symptom progression, and long-term outcome of the deficit syndrome in schizophrenia. *American Journal of Psychiatry*, **151**(3), 351–6.

Fioritti, A., Lo, R. L., and Melega, V. (1997) Reform said or done? The case of Emilia-Romagna within the Italian psychiatric context. *American Journal of Psychiatry*, **154**(1), 94–8.

Foucault, M. (1965) *Madness and civilisation: A history of insanity in the age of reason.* Random House Inc., New York.

Freudenberg, R. K., Bennett, D. H. , and May, A. R. (1957) The relative importance of physical and community methods in the treatment of schizophrenia, in *Report of Second International Congress of Psychiatry, Congress Report, 1.* Orell Fussli Arts Graphiques, Zurich, 157–78.

Fromm-Reichmann, F. (1948) Notes on the development of treatment of schizophrenics by psycho-analytic psychotherapy. *Psychiatry*, **11**, 263–70.

Gaebel, W., Frick, U., Kopcke, W., Linden, M., Muller, P., Muller-Spahn, F., et al. (1993) Early neuroleptic intervention in schizophrenia: are prodromal symptoms valid predictors of relapse? *British Journal of Psychiatry, Supplement no. 21*, 8–12.

Garety, P., Fowler, D., Kuipers, E., Freeman, D., Dunn, G., Bebbington, P., et al. (1997) London-East Anglia randomised controlled trial of cognitive-behavioural therapy for psychosis. II: Predictors of outcome. *British Journal of Psychiatry*, **171**, 420–6.

Garety, P. A., Kuipers, L., Fowler, D., Chamberlain, F., and Dunn, G. (1994) Cognitive behavioural therapy for drug-resistant psychosis. *British Journal of Medical Psychology*, **67**, 259–71.

Gelder, M. (1991) Adolf Meyer and his influence on British Psychiatry, in *150 years of British Psychiatry (1841–1991).* G. E. Berrios and H. Freeman, (ed.), Gaskell Press, London, 419–35.

Goffman, I. (1960) *Asylums: Essays on the social situation of mental patients and other inmates.* Penguin Books, Harmondsworth, Middlesex.

Goldberg, D. and Huxley, P. (1992) *Common mental disorders.* Routledge, London.

Gooch, C. and Leff, J. (1996) Factors affecting the success of community placement: the TAPS project 26. *Psychological Medicine*, **26**(3), 511–20.

Gournay, K. and Birley, J. (1998) Thorn: a new approach to mental health training, *Nursing Times*, **94**(49), 54–5.

Greenwood, N., Chisholm, B., Burns, T., and Harvey, K. (2000) Community mental health team caseloads and diagnostic case mix. *Psychiatric Bulletin*, **24**(8), 290–3.

Hafner, H., Behrens, S., De Vry, J., and Gattaz, W. F. (1991) An animal model for the effects of estradiol on dopamine-mediated behavior: implications for sex differences in schizophrenia. *Psychiatry Research*, **38**(2), 125–34.

Hafner, H., Maurer, K., Loffler, W., Fatkenheuer, B., an der, H. W., Riecher-Rossler, A., *et al.* (1994) The epidemiology of early schizophrenia. Influence of age and gender on onset and early course. *British Journal of Psychiatry, Supplement,* **164**(23), 29–38.

Harding, C. M., Brooks, G. W., Ashikaga, T., Strauss, J. S., and Breier, A. (1987) The Vermont longitudinal study of persons with severe mental illness, II: Long-term outcome of subjects who retrospectively met DSM-III criteria for schizophrenia. *American Journal of Psychiatry,* **144**(6), 727–35.

Harvey, K., Burns, T., Sedgwick, P., Higgitt, A., Creed, F., and Fahy, T. (2001) Relatives of patients with severe psychotic disorders: factors that influence contact frequency. Report from the UK700 trial. *British Journal of Psychiatry,* **178**, 248–54.

Hegarty, J. D., Baldessarini, R. J., Tohen, M., Waternaux, C., and Oepen, G. (1994) One hundred years of schizophrenia: a meta-analysis of the outcome literature. *American Journal of Psychiatry,* **151**(10), 1409–16.

Herman, J. L. (1992) Complex PTSD: A syndrome in survivors of prolonged and repeated trauma. *Journal of Traumatic Stress,* **5**(3), 377–91.

Hirsch, S., Bowen, J., Emami, J., Cramer, P., Jolley, A., Haw, C., *et al.* (1996) A one year prospective study of the effect of life events and medication in the aetiology of schizophrenic relapse. *British Journal of Psychiatry,* **168**(1), 49–56.

Hirsch, S. R., Gaind, R., Rohde, P. D., Stevens, B. C., and Wing, J. K. (1973) Outpatient maintenance of chronic schizophrenic patients with long-acting fluphenazine: double-blind placebo trial. Report to the Medical Research Council Committee on Clinical Trials in Psychiatry. *British Medical Journal,* **1**(854), 633–7.

Hirsch, S. R., Platt, S., Knights, A., and Weyman, A. (1979) Shortening hospital stay for psychiatric care: effect on patients and their families. *British Medical Journal,* **1**(6161), 442–6.

Hobbs, M., Mayou, R., Harrison, B., and Worlock, P. (1996) A randomised controlled trial of psychological debriefing for victims of road traffic accidents. *British Medical Journal,* **313**(7070), 1438–9.

Hogarty, G. E., Greenwald, D., Ulrich, R. F., Kornblith, S. J., DiBarry, A. L., Cooley, S., *et al.* (1997) Three-year trials of personal therapy among schizophrenic patients living with or independent of family, II: Effects on adjustment of patients. *American Journal of Psychiatry,* **154**(11), 1514–24.

Hogarty, G. E., Kornblith, S. J., Greenwald, D., DiBarry, A. L., Cooley, S., Flesher, S., *et al.* (1995) Personal therapy: a disorder-relevant psychotherapy for schizophrenia. *Schizophrenia Bulletin,* **21**(3), 379–93.

Holmes, T. H. and Rahe, R. H. (1967) The Social Readjustment Rating Scale. *Journal of Psychosomatic Research,* **11**(2), 213–18.

Hoult, J. (1986) Community care of the acutely mentally ill. *British Journal of Psychiatry,* **149**, 137–44.

Hoult, J., Reynolds, I., Charbonneau-Powis, M., Weekes, P., and Briggs, J. (1983) Psychiatric hospital versus community treatment: the results of a randomised trial. *Australian & New Zealand Journal of Psychiatry,* **17**(2), 160–7.

Hoult, J., Rosen, A., and Reynolds, I. (1984) Community orientated treatment compared to psychiatric hospital orientated treatment. *Social Science & Medicine,* **18**(11), 1005–10.

House of Commons Health Committee (2000) *Fourth Report: Provision of Mental Health Services, Volume I, Report and Proceedings of the Committee (373-I).* House of Commons, London.

Intagliata, J. (1982) Improving the quality of community care for the chronically mentally disabled: the role of case management. *Schizophrenia Bulletin,* **8**(4), 655–74.

Jackson, H., McGorry, P., Edwards, J., Hulbert, C., Henry, L., Francey, S., et al. (1998) Cognitively-oriented psychotherapy for early psychosis (COPE). Preliminary results. *British Journal of Psychiatry, Supplement,* **172**(33), 93–100.

James, P. and Burns, T. (2002) The influence of evidence on mental health care developments in the UK since 1980, in *Evidence in mental health care.* S. Priebe and M. Slade, eds. Brunner-Routledge, Hove and New York, 28–39.

Johnson, S. and Thornicroft, G. (1993) The sectorisation of psychiatric services in England and Wales. *Social Psychiatry & Psychiatric Epidemiology,* **28**(1), 45–7.

Johnson, S., Zinkler, M., and Priebe, S. (2001) Mental health service provision in England. *Acta Psychiatrica Scandinavica, Supplementum no.* 410, 47–55.

Jolley, A. G., Hirsch, S. R., Morrison, E., McRink, A., and Wilson, L. (1990) Trial of brief intermittent neuroleptic prophylaxis for selected schizophrenic outpatients: clinical and social outcome at two years. *British Medical Journal,* **301**(6756), 837–42.

Jones, D. (1982) The Borders Mental Health Service. *British Journal of Clinical & Social Psychiatry,* **2**, 8–12.

Jones, K. (1960) *Mental health and social policy.* Routledge & Kegan Paul, London.

Jones, K. and Poletti, A. (1985) Understanding the Italian Experience. *British Journal of Psychiatry,* **146**, 341–7.

Jones, M. (1952) *Social Psychiatry: A study of therapeutic communities.* Tavistock, London.

Jones, P., Rodgers, B., Murray, R., and Marmot, M. (1994) Child development risk factors for adult schizophrenia in the British 1946 birth cohort. *Lancet,* **344**(8934), 1398–1402.

Jorgensen, P. (1998) Early signs of psychotic relapse in schizophrenia. *British Journal of Psychiatry,* **172**, 327–30.

Jorm, A. F. (2000) Mental health literacy: Public knowledge and beliefs about mental disorders. *British Journal of Psychiatry,* **177**, 396–401.

Jorm, A. F., Angermeyer, M., and Katschnig, H. (2000) Public knowledge of and attitudes to mental disorders: a limiting factor in the optimal use of treatment services, in *Unmet Need in Psychiatry.* G. Andrews and A. S. Henderson, (ed.), Cambridge University Press, Cambridge, 399–413.

Jorm, A. F., Korten, A. E., Jacomb, P. A., Christensen, H., Rodgers, B., and Pollitt, P. (1997a) Public beliefs about causes and risk factors for depression and schizophrenia. *Social Psychiatry & Psychiatric Epidemiology,* **32**(3), 143–8.

Jorm, A. F., Korten, A. E., Rodgers, B., Pollitt, P., Jacomb, P. A., Christensen, H., et al. (1997b) Belief systems of the general public concerning the appropriate treatments for mental disorders. *Social Psychiatry Psychiatric Epidemiology,* **32**(8), 468–73.

Jorm, A. F., Korten, A. E., Jacomb, P. A., Rodgers, B., Pollitt, P., Christensen, H., et al. (1997c) Helpfulness of interventions for mental disorders: beliefs of health professionals compared with the general public. *British Journal of Psychiatry,* **171**, 233–7.

Katschnig, H. and Cooper, J. (1991) *Community Psychiatry.* Churchill Livingstone, Edinburgh.

Kemp, R., Kirov, G., Everitt, B., Hayward, P., and David, A. (1998) Randomised controlled trial of compliance therapy. 18-month follow-up. *British Journal of Psychiatry,* **172**(5), 413–19.

Kendler, K. S., Kessler, R. C., Walters, E. E., MacLean, C., Neale, M. C., Heath, A. C., et al. (1995) Stressful life events, genetic liability, and onset of an episode of major depression in women. *American Journal of Psychiatry,* **152**(6), 833–42.

Kendrick, T., Burns, T., Freeling, P., and Sibbald, B. (1994) Provision of care to general practice patients with disabling long-term mental illness: a survey in 16 practices. *British Journal of General Practice,* **44**(384), 301–5.

Kent, A. and Burns, T. (1996) Setting up an assertive community treatment service. *Advances in Psychiatric Treatment*, 2(4), 143–50.

Kielhofner, G., Mallinson, T., Crawford, C., Nowak, M., Rigby, M., Henry, A., *et al.* (1998) *A Users Manual for the Occupational Performance History Interview* (Version 2.0) *OPHI-II*. University of Illinois, Chicago.

Kingdon, D. G. and Turkington, D. (1994) *Cognitive-behavioural therapy for schizophrenia*. Guildford Press, New York.

Knapp, M., Beecham, J., Anderson, J., Dayson, D., Leff, J., Margolius, O., *et al.* (1990) The TAPS project. 3: Predicting the community costs of closing psychiatric hospitals. *British Journal of Psychiatry*, 157, 661–70.

Kosky, N. and Burns, T. (1995) Patient access to psychiatric records: Experience in an in-patient unit, *Psychiatric Bulletin*, 19, 87–90.

Kovess, V., Boisguerin, B., Antoine, D., and Reynauld, M. (1995) Has the sectorization of psychiatric services in France really been effective? *Social Psychiatry & Psychiatric Epidemiology*, 30(3), 132–8.

Kraepelin, E. (1919) *Dementia praecox and paraphrenia (Translated by Barclay, R.M.) Facsimile Edition*. 1971 Kreiger, New York.

Kuipers, L. and Bebbington, P. (1988) Expressed emotion research in schizophrenia: theoretical and clinical implications. *Psychological Medicine*, 18(4), 893–909.

Lacan, J. (1966) *Ecrits*. Le Seuil, Paris.

Laing, R. D. (1960) *The divided self*. Tavistock, London.

Lauber, C. and Rossler, W. (2001) [Early detection of schizophrenic psychoses]. *Schweizerische Rundschau fur Medizin Praxis*, 90(22), 987–92.

Leff, J. (1997) *Care in the Community: Illusion or Reality*. John Wiley & Sons, Chichester.

Leff, J. and Vaughn, C. (1981) The role of maintenance therapy and relatives' expressed emotion in relapse of schizophrenia: a two-year follow-up. *British Journal of Psychiatry*, 139, 102–4.

Lehman, A. F. (1995) Vocational rehabilitation in schizophrenia. *Schizophrenia Bulletin*, 21(4), 645–56.

Lehman, A. F., Goldberg, R., Dixon, L. B., McNary, S., Postrado, L., Hackman, A., *et al.* (2002) Improving employment outcomes for persons with severe mental illnesses. *Archives of General Psychiatry*, 59(2), 165–72.

Lehman, A. F. and Steinwachs, D. M. (1998) Translating research into practice: the Schizophrenia Patient Outcomes Research Team (PORT) treatment recommendations. *Schizophrenia Bulletin*, 24(1), 1–10.

Liberman, R. P., Hilty, D. M., Drake, R. E., and Tsang, H. W. (2001) Requirements for multidisciplinary teamwork in psychiatric rehabilitation. *Psychiatric Services*, 52(10), 1331–42.

Lidz, T. (1966) Adolf Meyer and the development of American psychiatry. *American Journal of Psychiatry*, 123, 320–32.

Lieberman, J. A., Alvir, J. M., Koreen, A., Geisler, S., Chakos, M., Sheitman, B., *et al.* (1996) Psychobiologic correlates of treatment response in schizophrenia. *Neuropsychopharmacology*, 14(3), (Suppl), 13S–21S.

Lindemann, E. (1944) Symptomatology and management of acute grief. *American Journal of Psychiatry*, 101, 141–8.

Loebel, A. D., Lieberman, J. A., Alvir, J. M., Mayerhoff, D. I., Geisler, S. H., and Szymanski, S. R. (1992) Duration of psychosis and outcome in first-episode schizophrenia. *American Journal of Psychiatry*, 149(9), 1183–8.

MacMillan, F. and Shiers, D. (2000) The IRIS Programme, in *Early Intervention in Psychosis*. M. Birchwood, D. Fowler, and C. Jackson, (ed.), John Wiley & Sons Ltd, New York, 315–26.

Main, T. F. (1946) The hospital as a therapeutic institution. *Bulletin of the Menninger Clinic*, **10**, 66–70.

Mangen, S. (1989) The politics of reform: origins and enactment of the Italian 'experience'. *International Journal of Social Psychiatry*, **35**(1), 7–20.

Mangen, S. P. (1985) Psychiatric policies: development and constraints, in *Mental Health Care in the European Community*. S. P. Mangen, (ed.), Croom Helm, London, 1–33.

Marder, S. R., Van Putten, T., Mintz, J., McKenzie, J., Lebell, M., Faltico, G., *et al.* (1984) Costs and benefits of two doses of fluphenazine. *Archives of General Psychiatry*, **41**(11), 1025–9.

Marder, S. R., Wirshing, W. C., Van Putten, T., Mintz, J., McKenzie, J., Johnston-Cronk, K., *et al.* (1994) Fluphenazine vs placebo supplementation for prodromal signs of relapse in schizophrenia. *Archives of General Psychiatry*, **51**(4), 280–7.

Mari, J. J. and Streiner, D. L. (1994) An overview of family interventions and relapse on schizophrenia: meta-analysis of research findings. *Psychological Medicine*, **24**(3), 565–78.

Marshall, M. and Lockwood, A. Assertive Community Treatment for people with severe mental disorders (Cochrane Review). The Cochrane Library [3]. 25-2-1998. Ref Type: Journal (Full)

Mayou, R. A., Ehlers, A., and Hobbs, M. (2000) Psychological debriefing for road traffic accident victims. Three-year follow-up of a randomised controlled trial. *British Journal of Psychiatry*, **176**, 589–93.

McCreadie, R. G., Phillips, K., Harvey, J. A., Waldron, G., Stewart, M., and Baird, D. (1991) The Nithsdale schizophrenia surveys. VIII: Do relatives want family intervention—and does it help? *British Journal of Psychiatry*, **158**, 110–13.

McFarlane, W. R., Lukens, E., Link, B., Dushay, R., Deakins, S. A., Newmark, M., *et al.* (1995) Multiple-family groups and psychoeducation in the treatment of schizophrenia. *Archives of General Psychiatry*, **52**(8), 679–87.

McGlashan, T. H., Levy, S. T., and Carpenter Jr., W. T., (1975) Integration and sealing over. Clinically distinct recovery styles from schizophrenia. *Archives of General Psychiatry*, **32**(10), 1269–72.

McGorry, P., Edwards, J. G., Mihalopoulos, C., Harrigan, S., and Jackson, H. J. (1996) EPPIC: an evolving system of early detection and optimal management. *Schizophrenia Bulletin*, **22**, 305–26.

McGorry, P. and Jackson, H. (1999) *Recognition and management of early psychosis. A preventative approach*. Cambridge University Press, Cambridge.

McGorry, P. D. (1994) The influence of illness duration on syndrome clarity and stability in functional psychosis: does the diagnosis emerge and stabilise with time? *Australian & New Zealand Journal of Psychiatry*, **28**(4), 607–19.

McGorry, P. D. and McConville, S. B. (1999) Insight in psychosis: an elusive target. *Comprehensive Psychiatry*, 40 (2), 131–42.

McGorry, P. D., Yung, A. R., Phillips, L. J., Yuen, H. P., Francey, S., Cosgrave, E. M., *et al.* (2002) Randomized controlled trial of interventions designed to reduce the risk of progression to first-episode psychosis in a clinical sample with subthreshold symptoms. *Archives of General Psychiatry*, **59**(10), 921–8.

McGuire, R., McCabe, R., and Priebe, S. (2001) Theoretical frameworks for understanding and investigating the therapeutic relationship in psychiatry. *Social Psychiatry & Psychiatric Epidemiology*, **36**(11), 557–64.

Millar, E., Garland, C., Ross, F., Kendrick, T., and Burns, T. (1999) Practice nurses and the care of patients receiving depot neuroleptic treatment: views on training, confidence and use of structured assessment. *Journal of Advanced Nursing*, **29**(6), 1454–61.

Minghella, E., Ford, R., Freeman, T., Hoult, J., McGlynn, P., and O'Halloran, P. (1998) *Open all hours: 24 hour response for people with mental health emergencies*. Sainsbury Centre for Mental Health, London.

Moore, S. (1960) A psychiatric out-patient nursing service. *Mental Health*, **20**, 54–4.

Mueser, K. T., Bond, G. R., Drake, R. E., and Resnick, S. G. (1998) Models of community care for severe mental illness: a review of research on case management. *Schizophrenia Bulletin*, **24**(1), 37–74.

National Association for Mental Health (1961) Emerging patterns for the mental health services and the public: Mental health is everybody's business. Proceedings of a conference held at Church House, Westminster, London, on 9th and 10th March 1961. Welbeck, Leeds.

National Institute for Mental Health in England. Early intervention for people with psychosis. Expert briefing. 2003. London, Department of Health.

Noffsinger, S. G. and Resnick, P. J. (1999) Violence and mental illness. *Current Opinion in Psychiatry*, **12**(6), 683–7.

O'Brien, A. and Firn, M. (2002) Clozapine initiation in the community. *Psychiatric Bulletin*, **26**, 339–41.

Onyett, S., Pillinger, T., and Muijen, M. (1997) Job satisfaction and burnout among members of community mental health teams. *Journal of Mental Health*, **6**(1), 55–66.

Overall, J. E. and Gorham, D. L. (1962) The Brief Psychiatric Rating Scale. *Psychological Reports*, **10**, 799–812.

Pai, S. and Kapur, R. L. (1981) The burden on the family of a psychiatric patient: development of an interview schedule. *British Journal of Psychiatry*, **138**, 332–5.

Pasamanick, B., Scarpitti, F. R., and Leyton, M. (1964) Home versus hospital care for schizophrenics. *Journal of the American Medical Association*, **187**, 177–81.

Paykel, E. S. (1978) Contribution of life events to causation of psychiatric illness. *Psychological Medicine*, **8**(2), 245–53.

Paykel, E. S. (1997) The interview for recent life events. *Psychological Medicine*, **27**(2), 301–10.

Perry, A., Tarrier, N., Morriss, R., McCarthy, E., and Limb, K. (1999) Randomised controlled trial of efficacy of teaching patients with bipolar disorder to identify early symptoms of relapse and obtain treatment. *British Medical Journal*, **318**, 149–53.

Pilling, S., Bebbington, P., Kuipers, E., Garety, P., Geddes, J., Orbach, G., *et al.* (2002) Psychological treatments in schizophrenia: I. Meta-analysis of family intervention and cognitive behaviour therapy. *Psychological Medicine*, **32**(5), 763–82.

Poulton, R., Caspi, A., Moffitt, T. E., Cannon, M., Murray, R., and Harrington, H. (2000) Children's self-reported psychotic symptoms and adult schizophreniform disorder: a 15-year longitudinal study. *Archives of General Psychiatry*, **57**(11), 1053–8.

Priebe, S. and Gruyters, T. (1993) The role of the helping alliance in psychiatric community care. A prospective study. *Journal of Nervous & Mental Disease*, **181**(9), 552–7.

Querido, A. (1968) *The development of socio-medical care in the Netherlands*. Routledge and Kegan Paul, London.

Raphael, B. and Meldrum, L. (1995) Does debriefing after psychological trauma work? *British Medical Journal*, 310(6993), 1479–80.

Rapoport, R. N. (1960) *Community as doctor*. Tavistock, London.

Ratcliffe, R. A. W. (1962) The open door: ten years' experience in Dingleton. *Lancet*, **ii**, 188–90.

Ritchie, J. H. (1994) The report of the enquiry into the care and treatment of Christopher Clunis presented to the Chairman of the North East Thames and South East Thames Regional Health Authorities. HMSO, London.

Rollinick, S., Heather, N., and Bell, A. (1992) Negotiating behaviour change in medical settings: the development of brief motivational interviewing. *Journal of Mental Health*, **1**, 25–37.

Royal College of Psychiatrists (2000) *Community Care*. Royal College of Psychiatrists, London, College Report 86.

Ryle, A. and Kerr, I. B. (2002) *Introducing Cognitive Analytic Therapy: Principles and Practice* Wiley, Chichester.

Sandler, J., Dare, C., and Holder, A. (1992) *The patient and the analyst.* (2nd edn). H Karnac, London.

Schene, A. H., Tessler, R. C., and Gamache, G. M. (1994) Instruments measuring family or caregiver burden in severe mental illness. *Social Psychiatry & Psychiatric Epidemiology,* **29**(5), 228–40.

Shapiro, F. and Maxfield, L. (2002) Eye movement desensitization and reprocessing (EMDR): Information processing in the treatment of trauma. *Journal of Clinical Psychology,* **58**(8), 933–46.

Simpson, G. M. and Angus, J. W. (1970) A rating scale for extrapyramidal side effects. *Acta Psychiatrica Scandinavica Supplement,* **212**, 11–19.

Singh, S. P., Wright, C., Burns, T., Joyce, E., and Barnes, T., (2003) Developing early intervention services in the NHS: a survey to guide workforce and training needs. *Psychiatric Bulletin,* **27**, 254–8.

Slade, M., Powell, R., Rosen, A., and Strathdee, G. (2000) Threshold Assessment Grid (TAG): the development of a valid and brief scale to assess the severity of mental illness. *Social Psychiatry & Psychiatric Epidemiology,* **35**(2), 78–85.

Sledge, W. H., Tebes, J., and Rakfeldt, J. (1995) Acute crisis respite care, in *Emergency mental health services in the community.* M. Phelan, G. Strathdee, and G. Thornicroft, (ed.), Cambridge University Press, Cambridge.

Smyth, M. G. and Hoult, J. (2000) The home treatment enigma. *British Medical Journal,* **320**(7230), 305–9.

Snowden, P. (2002) Who should outreach? *Journal of Forensic Psychiatry,* **13**(1), 167–87.

Solomon, P. (1992) The efficacy of case management services for severely mentally disabled clients. *Community Mental Health Journal,* **28**(3), 163–80.

Solomon, P. and Draine, J. (1995*a*) One-year outcomes of a randomized trial of case management with seriously mentally ill clients leaving jail. *Evaluation Review,* **19**, 256–73.

Solomon, P. and Draine, J. (1995*b*) The efficacy of a consumer case management team: 2-year outcomes of a randomized trial. *Journal of Mental Health Administration,* **22**(2), 135–46.

Steadman, H. J., Mulvey, E. P., Monahan, J., Robbins, P. C., Appelbaum, P. S., Grisso, T., *et al.* (1998) Violence by people discharged from acute psychiatric inpatient facilities and by others in the same neighbourhoods. *Archives of General Psychiatry,* **55**(5), 393–401.

Stefansson, C. G. and Cullberg, J. (1986) Introducing community mental health services. The effects on a suburban patient population. *Acta Psychiatrica Scandinavica,* **74**(4), 368–78.

Stein, L. I. and Santos, A. B. (1998) *Assertive Community Treatment of Persons with Severe Mental Illness.* WW Norton & Company Inc, New York.

Stein, L. I. and Test, M. A. (1980) Alternative to mental hospital treatment. I. Conceptual model, treatment program, and clinical evaluation. *Archives of General Psychiatry,* **37**(4), 392–7.

Strathdee, G. (1998) Deploying a CMHT for the effective care of individuals with schizophrenia, in *Acute psychosis, schizophrenia and co-morbid disorders,* A. Lee, (ed.), Gaskell, London.

Strathdee, G. and Williams, P. (1984) A survey of psychiatrists in primary care: the silent growth of a new service. *Journal of the Royal College of General Practitioners,* **34**, 615–18.

Summerfield, D. (1999) A critique of seven assumptions behind psychological trauma programmes in war-affected areas. *Social Science & Medicine,* **48**, 1449–62.

Summerfield, D. (2001) The invention of post-traumatic stress disorder and the social usefulness of a psychiatric category. *British Medical Journal,* **322**(7278), 95–8.

Szasz, T. S. (1972) *The myth of mental illness: Foundations of a theory of personal conduct.* Paladin, London.

Szmukler, G. I., Burgess, P., Herrman, H., Benson, A., Colusa, S., and Bloch, S. (1996) Caring for relatives with serious mental illness: the development of the Experience of Caregiving Inventory. *Social Psychiatry & Psychiatric Epidemiology*, **31**(3–4), 137–48.

Szmukler, G. I., Wykes, T., and Parkman, S. (1998) Care-giving and the impact on carers of a community mental health service. PRiSM Psychosis Study 6. *British Journal of Psychiatry*, **173**, 399–403.

Talbott, J. A., Clark, G. H. J., Sharfstein, S. S., and Klein, J. (1987) Issues in developing standards governing psychiatric practice in community mental health centers. *Hospital & Community Psychiatry*, **38**(11), 1198–202.

Tansella, M. (1987) Editorial: the Italian experience and its implications. *Psychological Medicine*, **17**, 283–9.

Taylor, P. J. and Gunn, J. (1999) Homicides by people with mental illness: Myth and Reality. *British Journal of Psychiatry*, **174**, 9–14.

Teague, G. B., Bond, G. R., and Drake, R. E. (1998) Program fidelity in assertive community treatment: development and use of a measure. *American Journal of Orthopsychiatry*, **68**(2), 216–32.

Trauer, T., Callaly, T., Hantz, P., Little, J., Shields, R., and Smith, J. (1999) Health of the Nation Outcome Scales. Results of the Victorian field trial. *British Journal of Psychiatry*, **174**, 380–8.

Turton, N. (2001) Welfare benefits and work disincentives. *Journal of Mental Health*, **10**(3), 285–300.

Van Etten, M. L. and Taylor, S. (1998) Comparative efficacy of treatments for post-traumatic stress disorder: a meta-analysis. *Clinical Psychology and Psychotherapy*, **5**, 126–44.

Volovik, V. M. and Zachepitskii, R. A. (1986) Treatment, care, and rehabilitation of the chronic mentally ill in the USSR. *Hospital & Community Psychiatry*, **37**(3), 280–2.

Warner, J. P., King, M., Blizard, R., McClenahan, Z., and Tang, S. (2000) Patient-held shared care records for individuals with mental illness: Randomised controlled evaluation. *British Journal of Psychiatry*, **177**, 319–24.

Weisbrod, B. A., Test, M. A., and Stein, L. I. (1980) Alternative to mental hospital treatment. II. Economic benefit-cost analysis. *Archives of General Psychiatry*, **37**(4), 400–5.

Weissman, M. M. and Markowitz, J. C. (1994) Interpersonal psychotherapy. Current status. *Archives of General Psychiatry*, **51**(8), 599–606.

Wessely, S., Rose, S., and Bisson, J. (1998) *A systematic review of brief psychological interventions (debriefing) for the treatment of immediate trauma related symptoms and the prevention of post traumatic stress disorder*. Cochrane Library, 4. Update Software, Oxford.

Wilkinson, G., Piccinelli, M., Falloon, I., Krekorian, H., and McLees, S. (1995) An evaluation of community-based psychiatric care for people with treated long-term mental illness. *British Journal of Psychiatry*, **167**(1), 26–37.

Willetts, L. E. and Leff, J. (1997) Expressed emotion and schizophrenia: the efficacy of a staff training programme. *Journal of Advanced Nursing*, **26**(6), 1125–33.

Willson, M. (1987) *Occupational therapy in long term psychiatry*. Churchill Livingstone, Edinburgh.

Wing, J., Curtis, R. H., and Beevor, A. (1999) Health of the Nation Outcome Scales (HoNOS). Glossary for HoNOS score sheet. *British Journal of Psychiatry*, **174**, 432–4.

Wing, J. K., Cooper, J. E., and Sartorius, N. (1974) *The measurement and classification of psychiatric symptoms: An instruction manual for the PSE and the Catego Program*. Cambridge University Press, Cambridge.

Wolff, G., Pathare, S., Craig, T., and Leff, J. (1996a) Community knowledge of mental illness and reaction to mentally ill people. *British Journal of Psychiatry*, **168**(2), 191–8.

Wolff, G., Pathare, S., Craig, T., and Leff, J. (1996b) Community attitudes to mental illness. *British Journal of Psychiatry*, **168**(2), 183–90.

Wood, H. and Carr, S. (1998) *Locality services in mental health, developing home treatment and assertive outreach: The North Birmingham Experience.* Sainsbury Centre for Mental Health, London.

Wooff, K. and Goldberg, D. P. (1988) Further observations on the practice of community care in Salford. Differences between community psychiatric nurses and mental health social workers. *British Journal of Psychiatry*, **153**, 30–7.

Wooff, K., Goldberg, D. P., and Fryers, T. (1988) The practice of community psychiatric nursing and mental health social work in Salford. Some implications for community care. *British Journal of Psychiatry*, **152**, 783–92.

World Health Organization (1992) *The ICD-10 Classification of Mental and Behavioural Disorders.* World Health Organization, Geneva.

Wright, C., Catty, J., Burns, T., and Watt, H. (2000) Classification and sustainability of home treatment for mental health problems. *British Journal of Psychiatry*, In preparation.

Wright, C., Burns, T., James, P., Billings, J., Johnson, S., Muijen, M., *et al.* (2003) Assertive outreach teams in London: models of operation. Pan-London Assertive Outreach Study, Part 1. *British Journal of Psychiatry*, **183**, 132–8.

Zubin, J. and Spring, B. (1977) Vulnerability – a new view of schizophrenia. *Journal of Abnormal Psychology*, **86**(2), 103–26.

Index

Lightning Source UK Ltd.
Milton Keynes UK
15 February 2010

150106UK00005B/1/A